Carcinogens and Mutagens in the Environment

Volume III
Naturally Occurring Compounds:
Epidemiology and Distribution

Editor

Hans F. Stich, Ph.D.
Head
Environmental Carcinogenesis Unit
British Columbia Cancer Research Centre
Professor of Zoology
University of British Columbia
Vancouver, British Columbia, Canada

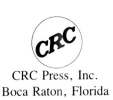

CRC Press, Inc.
Boca Raton, Florida

Library of Congress Cataloging in Publication Data
(Revised for volumes 2 and 3)

Main entry under title:

Carcinogens and mutagens in the environment.

Includes bibliographies and indexes.
Contents: v. 1. Food products — v. 2. Naturally
occurring compounds: endogenous formation and
modulation — v. 3. Naturally occurring compounds:
epidemiology and distribution.
1. Carcinogens. 2. Mutagens. 3. Environ-
mentally induced diseases. I. Stich, H. F.
(Hans F.), 1927-   [DNLM: 1. Carcinogens,
Environmental. 2. Mutagens. 3. Environmental
pollutants. QZ 202 C2651]
RC268.6.C365   616.99'4071   81-21764
ISBN 0-8493-5881-7 (v. 1)

Direct all inquiries to CRC Press, Inc., 2000 Corporate Blvd., N.W., Boca Raton, Florida, 33431.

© 1983 by CRC Press, Inc.

International Standard Book Number 0-8493-5882-5 (Volume II)
International Standard Book Number 0-8493-5883-3 (Volume III)

Library of Congress Card Number 81-21764
Printed in the United States

PREFACE

Daily each member of the human population ingests, inhales, or comes into contact in other ways with thousands of chemicals, including carcinogens, mutagens, and teratogens. The individual is constantly bombarded by news that one or more of the most cherished food items is hazardous to health. Regulatory agencies face the difficulty each day of making decisions on the basis of totally inadequate scientific data. It is therefore not surprising to find a frightened public, irritated industrialists, pressed civil servants, and underpaid scientists clamoring for more data on human populations and larger influence in the decision-making process that may affect everyone's lives.

Our lack of understanding of environmental toxicology becomes only too evident from the observation that we cannot even guess about the relative contribution of man-made agents and naturally occurring chemicals to the total carcinogenic or mutagenic load in a particular environment. The information available to assess a particular hazard to human health is shockingly inadequate when we consider the millions of chemicals in our environment, the few thousand chemicals tested for genotoxicity, and the paltry hundred or so compounds that have been properly evaluated for their carcinogenicity and teratogenicity. The difficulties involved in trying to assess the carcinogenic and genotoxic load will be further compounded when testing programs are extended to complex mixtures. The carcinogenicity and genotoxicity of a complex mixture does not seem to be a simple sum of the activities of the individual compounds because of a multitude of synergistic, antagonistic, co-carcinogenic, and co-mutagenic interactions between its various components.

Moreover, the composition of any mixture when ingested or inhaled will be subject to continuous change within the body that will in turn affect its carcinogenic and genotoxic potential. Finally, the testing of combinations and permutations between only a few compounds would rapidly exhaust the total available manpower and funding of an entire nation. A simple calculation reveals that the testing of all permutations between 10 different chemicals would lead to about 10 million possible permutations, $1\frac{1}{2}$ billion dishes, approximately 79 million working hours, and 9.8×10^9 U.S. dollars when the Ames' Salmonella mutagenicity test is used on 5 strains, at 5 doses, and with or without S9 activation. With 20 different compounds, the number of man years would amount to approximately 3.3×10^{16} and the cost to 6.5×10^{21} U.S. dollars. These are staggering figures considering that 20 compounds is a relatively small number when we realize that 2000 or more chemicals are found, for example, in such widely consumed beverages as coffee and tea. In spite of these and other apparently insurmountable difficulties, the search for solutions will and must continue. The papers in this volume are an example of this effort.

H.F. Stich

THE EDITOR

Hans F. Stich, Ph.D., is Head, Environmental Carcinogenesis Unit, British Columbia Cancer Research Centre and Professor in the Department of Zoology and in the Department of Pathology, University of British Columbia, Vancouver, B. C., Canada.

Dr. Stich received his Ph.D. in Developmental Biology in 1949 from Faculty of Arts and Science at the University of Wurzburg, Germany. He also studied tropical medicine at the same university.

He is a member of the Environmental Contaminants Advisory Committee on Mutagenesis, Health and Welfare Canada; a Director of the British Columbia Cancer Foundation; Professional Consultant of the B.C. Cancer Control Agency; Councilor of the Environment Mutagen Society; on the editorial board of *Mutation Research* and *Cancer Research*; was chairman of the Grant Panel on Environment Toxicology; and Chairman of the Grant Panel on Cell Biology and Genetics of the Natural Science and Engineering Research Council Canada.

Dr. Stich has presented numerous invited lectures at international and national meetings as well as guest lectures at various universities and institutes. He has published over 180 papers to date. His major research interests include the etiology of oral and esophageal carcinomas among betel nut and tobacco chewers, the use of genotoxicity tests to detect naturally occurring carcinogens in food products and beverages, and the assessment of a mutagenic load by examining the synergistic and antagonistic interactions between mutagens, co-mutagens, and antimutagens.

CONTRIBUTORS

Michael J. Ashwood-Smith, Ph.D.
Professor
Department of Biology
University of Victoria
Victoria, British Columbia, Canada

Helmut Bartsch, Ph.D.
Head
Unit of Environmental Carcinogens and
  Host Factors
International Agency for Research on
  Cancer
Lyon, France

Bruce A. Bohm, Ph.D.
Professor
Botany Department
University of British Columbia
Vancouver, British Columbia, Canada

Kamalesh Chatterjee, Ph.D.
Associate Professor
Department of Zoology
School of Life Sciences
North Eastern Hill University
Shillong, India

Nicholas E. Day, Ph.D.
Head
Unit of Biostatistics
International Agency for Research on
  Cancer
Lyon, France

Marlin Friesen, Ph.D.
Scientist
Unit of Environmental Carcinogens and
  Host Factors
International Agency for Research on
  Cancer
Lyon, France

Waltraud Göggelmann, Dr. rer. nat.
Institut für Toxikologie und Biochemie
Gesellschaft für Strahlen-und
  Umweltforschung
Munich, West Germany

Iwao Hirono, M.D.
Professor
Department of Carcinogenesis and
  Cancer Susceptibility
Institute of Medical Science
University of Tokyo
Tokyo, Japan

J.H.C. Ho, M.D., D.Sc.
Medical and Health Department
Institute of Radiology and Oncology
Queen Elizabeth Hospital
Kowloon, Hong Kong

Philip K. Hopke, Ph.D.
Professor of Environmental
  Chemistry
Institute for Environmental Studies
University of Illinois
Urbana, Illinois

Dolly P. Huang, Ph.D.
Scientific Officer
Medical and Health Department
Institute of Radiology and Oncology
Queen Elizabeth Hospital
Kowloon, Hong Kong

Tsuneo Kada, D.Sc.
Head
Department of Induced Mutation
National Institute of Genetics
Mishima, Japan

Sigetosi Kamiyama, M.D.
Professor
Department of Hygiene
Akita University School of Medicine
Akita, Japan

Govind J. Kapadia, Ph.D.
Professor
College of Pharmacy and Pharmacal
  Sciences
Howard University
Washington, D.C.

Christian Malaveille, Dr.-Ing.
Scientist
Unit of Environmental Carcinogens and
  Host Factors
International Agency for Research on
  Cancer
Lyon, France

Osamu Michioka, Ph.D.
Research Associate
Department of Hygiene
Akita University School of Medicine
Akita, Japan

A.B. Miller, M.B., F.R.C.P.(C)
Director
NCIC Epidemiology Unit
University of Toronto
Toronto, Ontario, Canada

Julia F. Morton, D.Sc.
Director
Morton Collectanea
Research Professor of Biology
University of Miami
Coral Gables, Florida

Howard F. Mower, Ph.D.
Professor
Department of Biochemistry and
  Biophysics
John A. Burns School of Medicine
University of Hawaii at Manoa
Honolulu, Hawaii

Kazuko Namiki, Ph.D.
Professor
Sugiyama Women's University
Nagoya, Japan

Mitsuo Namiki, Ph.D.
Professor
Department of Food Science and
  Technology
Nagoya University
Nagoya, Japan

Earle Nestmann, Ph.D.
Research Scientist
Mutagenesis Section
Environmental Health Directorate
Health and Welfare Canada
Ottawa, Ontario, Canada

Toshihiko Osawa, Ph.D.
Assistant Professor
Department of Food Science and
  Technology
Nagoya University
Nagoya, Japan

Michael J. Plewa, Ph.D.
Associate Professor of Genetics
Institute for Environmental Studies
University of Illinois
Urbana, Illinois

Gerald A. Poulton, Ph.D., F.C.I.C.
Associate Professor
Department of Chemistry
University of Victoria
Victoria, British Columbia, Canada

G. Subba Rao, Ph.D.
Director and Chief Research Scientist
Division of Biochemistry
Head
Laboratory of Pharmacology
  Research Institute
American Dental Association Health
  Foundation
Chicago, Illinois

J.L. Sailo, Ph.D.
Medical Officer
North Eastern Hill University
Shillong, India

Richard H.C. San, Ph.D.
Chief
Carcinogen Testing Laboratory
British Columbia Cancer Research
  Centre
Assistant Professor
Department of Medical Genetics
University of British Columbia
Vancouver, British Columbia, Canada

D.R. Stoltz, D.V.M.
Research Scientist
Toxicology Research Division
Bureau of Chemical Safety
Food Directorate
Health Protection Branch
Health and Welfare Canada
Ottawa, Ontario, Canada

Peter Spitzauer, Dr. rer. nat.
Lehrstühl für Ökologische Chemie der
 TU München
Freising-Weihenstephan, West Germany

Bela Toth, D.V.M.
Professor
Eppley Institute for Research in Cancer
 and Allied Diseases
University of Nebraska Medical Center
Omaha, Nebraska

Keiichi Tsuji, Ph.D.
Senior Scientist
Institute of Physical and Chemical
 Research
Toshimaku, Japan

TABLE OF CONTENTS

Part I
Epidemiological Evidence

Chapter 1

HERBAL TEA CONSUMPTION AND ESOPHAGEAL CANCER

Govind J. Kapadia, G. Subba Rao, and Julia F. Morton

TABLE OF CONTENTS

I. INTRODUCTION

Although carcinoma of the esophagus is a comparatively rare form of cancer, it is one of the most difficult ones to diagnose in the early stage.[1,2] Once this relatively slow-growing type of tumor (predominantly squamous, rarely basal) is diagnosed, prognosis is usually poor since the overall long-term survival rate is below 2%. Thus, there is general belief that the best chance of combatting esophageal cancer is through prevention rather than treatment.[1-3]

The epidemiological evidence for the occurrence of a number of clearly defined geographical areas with a remarkably high incidence of esophageal cancer (Figure 1) has generated active research in the search for its cause(s). This has resulted in noteworthy correlation between the usage of native plant products and esophageal cancer zones on a worldwide basis. Among these, perhaps the most significant one is the potential causal relationship between consumption of herbal teas and incidence of this cancer. The use of herbal teas is rapidly gaining acceptance in Western countries thanks to the current ''back-to-nature'' movement which advocates ''if it is natural, it should be good.'' A review of herbal teas, their cancer-causing potential, and its significance in combatting what appears to be a preventable form of cancer, are presented in this chapter.

II. HERBAL TEAS USED AS BEVERAGES AND STIMULANTS

A. Commonly Used Teas

Common or ordinary tea consists of leaves and leaf buds of *Camellia sinensis* Kuntze (Theaceae). Black tea is prepared by heaping the fresh leaves and buds in a damp area until fermentation has begun, then rapidly drying with artificial heat and mechanical means. The tea leaves turn dark because of oxidation. Green tea is prepared by briefly steaming, partially drying, then rapidly firing the freshly picked leaves in copper pans or drums over a mild artificial heat, a process that causes little oxidation and thus retains the green color. Black tea has a strong flavor but green tea contains more polyphenols and releases caffeine more quickly in the infusion.

Several epidemiological surveys conducted around the world suggest a strong association between the observed high incidence of esophageal cancer and the excessive consumption of common tea.[4-9] Recent animal studies suggest that the carcinogenicity of tea is attributable to its tannin content, e.g., condensed catechin tannin, now termed proanthocyanidin.[10] There is a wide variation in tannin content of commonly used teas which could be as low as 4% in some green teas and as high as 33% in black tea. The cultivar and stage of growth of plucked leaves affect the tannin level;[11] the bud and the first leaf may have 26.5 and 25.9%, respectively, while the third leaf only 17.1%.

It is believed that drinking tea with milk renders the tannin inactive through the binding action of protein. Historians allege that tea was regarded only as a therapeutic brew in China until the 6th Century A.D. As a beverage, the Chinese prefer a nonastringent, low-tannin tea. Dutch traders carried tea to Europe in 1610, but in England in 1660 it was still classed as a medicinal product and physicians viewed it as harmful. The British adopted tea as a beverage only after they started putting milk in it. Medical authorities realized then and continued to assert that tannin is detrimental. The following is a passage from the 1923 edition of the British Pharmaceutical Codex:

''The properties of tannin depend upon its chemical interaction with protein or gelatine. When taken by mouth it gives the characteristic property of astringency, coagulates the protein material surrounding the epithelium, and even penetrates some of the superficial cells.''

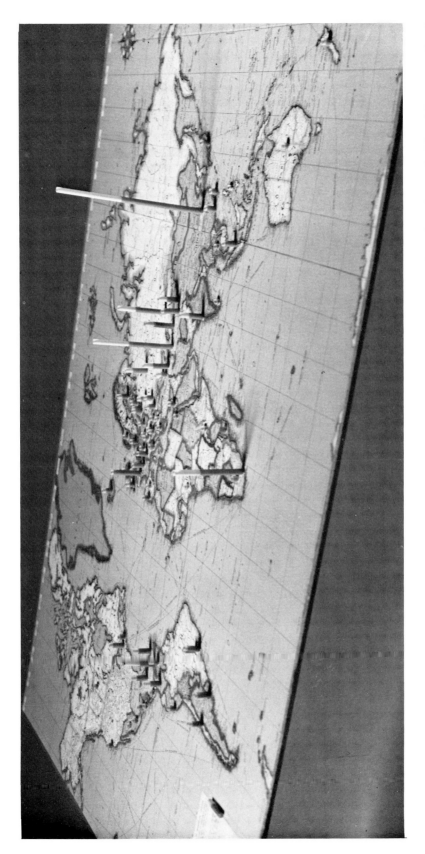

FIGURE 1.   The occurrence of esophageal cancer in relation to geographical location.   Photograph of a three-dimensional world map bar graph with each bar representing the annual rate of esophageal cancer in a specific geographic location per 200,000 persons, all ages, age-standardized.   The dark portion of each bar shows the annual rate per 100,000 men; the light portion shows the annual rate per 100,000 women.   The map dimension, 118 × 76 cm; scale, 1 mm = 1 person per year.

Thus, carcinoma of the esophagus is rare among the British who still put milk in their tea, while it was very common among the Dutch about 100 years ago, when they drank tea regularly without milk. When the Dutch switched from tea to coffee as the national beverage, the disease became very rare.[12] Currently, in England there is concern because of the modern mode of dispensing the working man's tea-break "cupper" through a vending machine. The tea is powdered instant tea and reportedly higher in tannin than the instant product made in America. It is vended along with powdered non-dairy creamer (or "whitener") which contains little or no protein to bind the tannin.[13] The usual amount of milk (about a tablespoonful) adds about 650 mg of protein to a cup of tea.

In all of the above-mentioned surveys, tea was taken as a hot drink and excessive heat was suspected as a carcinogenic factor rather than the tea.[4] Interestingly, there is no such disease link with the use of exceedingly hot coffee and, wherever the rate of esophageal cancer is alarming, it is the middle third of the esophagus that is most often affected rather than the upper third, which is more exposed to heat. Further, there is at least one well-substantiated case of an individual who drank only strong iced tea without milk (3, 4, or more glasses every day), avoided coffee, never used tobacco, indulged very little in spirits, and died of esophageal cancer at the age of 53.[14] Similarly, in another case, an American soldier took up tea drinking while with the U.S. Army in Korea. After his return home, he took a large thermos of tea, without milk, to work every day. During the winter, he would also drink tea at home in the evening. He, too, succumbed to esophageal cancer at the age of 46.

The 1975 epidemiological survey suggested a strong correlation between esophageal cancer and the consumption of tea-rice-gruel at least 3 times a week in the high-risk provinces of Japan.[7] This finding was recently confirmed by a 10-year follow-up study which showed an extra risk in drinking tea in addition to eating tea-rice-gruel.[9] The cancer-promoting effect of tea has been demonstrated in skin-painting tests with mice.[15,16] In the authors' laboratories, the tannin fraction from tea shipped from a plantation in Assam, India produced tumors at the injection site in 26 of 30 animals (NIH black rats) tested.[10]

The tannin/cancer correlation is strengthened by the fact that the betel nut (*Areca catechu* L.), which contains 14.9 to 18.0% catechin tannin,[17] has been linked repeatedly to esophageal and oral cancer — whether eaten or chewed, and with or without lime or tobacco leaf in the quid.[14,18] An extract of betel nut alone has produced tumors at the injection site in 100% of the rats used in the authors' studies.[19] Oral and gastric lesions and carcinomas in hamsters have resulted from exposure to the polyphenolic fraction of betel nuts either alone or with lime and tobacco.[20]

Furthermore, a hospital study in Djibouti revealed that esophageal cancer is prevalent there only among the various ethnic populations who habitually chew the leaves and twigs of khat, or so-called Abyssinian tea, *Catha edulis* Forsk, ex Endl. (Celastraceae).[21] The leaves of khat contain as much as 14% condensed catechin tannin.[22]

B. Less Commonly Used Teas

Many indigenous plants served as local beverages long before the worldwide exploitation of the common tea *(C. sinensis)*. Others have been adopted as substitutes for common tea when the latter was unobtainable. Epidemiological data on this group of teas are generally not available. However, because of the detection of one or more known chemical carcinogens in these teas, their usage has been implicated in the incidence of esophageal as well as other forms of cancer.

South American maté, or matté — the dried and often toasted leaves of *Ilex paraguariensis* St. Hil. (Aquifoliaceae), produced mainly in Argentina and Brazil — has been found to contain 9.1 to 12.4% tannin and 1.7 to 1.2% caffeine as well. It is especially favored by the gauchos of Rio Grande do Sul, southern Brazil, who steep it for a prolonged period, and that region is precisely Brazil's area of highest risk for esophageal cancer.[23]

The dried young leaves of cassena, or Carolina tea, *Ilex vomitoria* Ait. (Aquifoliaceae), have long been utilized for beverage purposes in coastal South Carolina, and about 50 years ago there were two attempts to commercialize cultivation and processing but the product could not compete successfully with imported maté.[24]

Ayapana, *Eupatorium triplinerve* Vahl (Asteraceae), a resinous subshrub native to Brazil, has been widely cultivated and naturalized in the tropics. In 1826, the dried leaves were being shipped to France from the island of Bourbon, the infusion being prescribed as a febrifuge and much consumed in that country (as well as on the Caribbean island of St. Thomas) as a substitute for tea. The plant contains the sesquiterpene hydrocarbon, β-selinene and coumarin, which is carcinogenic.[25] The decoction is highly astringent and a potent remedy for diarrhea and dysentery which are indicative of its high tannin content and thus a potential threat to the esophagus.[26]

Throughout the southern U.S., the young root of sassafras, *Sassafras albidum* Nees (Lauraceae), is commonly chewed and is also boiled, fresh or dried, for "tea" which is used as a beverage as well as for medicinal purposes. Aromatic oil derived from the sassafras root bark consisting mainly (70 to 90%) of safrole was formerly much utilized in flavoring confections, soft drinks, and pharmaceutical products. Such use was banned by the U.S. Food and Drug Administration in 1960 after safrole was found to be hepatocarcinogenic in the rat.[27] Dihydrosafrole has induced esophageal tumors in rats.[28] There has been much concern expressed because of the wide marketing of the chipped sassafras root bark for use as "tea". However, some investigators have found a high percentage of low-safrole wood chips mixed with the bark and because of the insolubility of safrole in water, such sassafras tea, prepared from inferior material, appears to be relatively safe for ingestion.[29]

Fragrant or sweet goldenrod, *Solidago odora* Air. (Asteraceae), grows wild from New England to Texas. In pioneer days, dried leaves and flowers were sold for use as tea, the assumption being that both were innocuous as well as agreeable. The essential oil of the leaves has the odor of sassafras and anise combined, therefore, chemical study is needed to determine if safrole is present and how much might be ingested with the tea.

III. HERBAL TEAS USED FOR MEDICINAL PURPOSES

Although the use of herbal teas for medicinal purposes dates back to primitive cultures, this practice continues to flourish to this date in both Old and New World countries. The number of these teas is obviously very large because each culture and ethnic group appears to have made selections for various reasons, the prime criterion being local availability. People use what they have. Only a limited number of epidemiological surveys attempting to correlate their usage with the incidence of cancer is currently available. Of these, the three recent surveys of esophageal cancer victims on the island of Curacao (in the Caribbean), in the Coro region of northwestern Venezuela, and the Low Country of South Carolina in the U.S., suggest a causal relationship between the usage of certain tannin-rich herbal teas for medicinal/beverage purposes and the cancer incidences.[12,14,24,30] Table 1 summarizes suspect plants, the area of use, and the results of carcinogenic bioassays with various extracts/constituents of the plants.

IV. HERBAL TEAS CURRENTLY SOLD IN HEALTH FOOD STORES

The modern health food stores in the U.S., Canada, and in most European countries offer an amazing array of natural products of plant origin to the unsuspecting public. Within the past few years, there appears to have emerged a booming business in herbal teas. Many of these are offered as caffeine-free substitutes for common tea, but in most cases their chemical composition is not revealed. Some packaged "teas" contain the dried material (leaves/stems/bark/roots) of a single species and the botanical name may appear on the label. Others may

Table 1

HERBAL TEAS USED FOR MEDICINAL PURPOSES IN HIGH-RISK AREAS FOR ESOPHAGEAL CANCER

Plant species (family)	Locality	Use[a]	Known chemical constituents	Carcinogenic bioassay (including references in parentheses)
Acacia glauca Moench, formerly *A. villosa* Willd. (Leguminosae)	Curacao	Root decoction gargled for sore throat, to loosen phlegm; also to "ripen a tumor" in the throat	Tannin	Fibrosarcomas at injection site in 100% of rats, root extract, s.c. dosing (37,38). Atypical papilloma in esophagus of 14% hamsters, pulverized plant with corn starch in cheek pouch (39).
Annona muricata L. (Annonaceae)	Curacao, other Caribbean Islands, Bahamas	Leaf decoction as bush tea, often drunk daily; for asthma, kidney, or gallbladder ailments, hypertension; to infants as soporific	Tannin	Fibrosarcomas at injection site in 33% rats, leaf extract, s.c. dosing. Carcinoma in cheek pouch in 25% of hamsters, pulverized leaves (39).
Chenopodium ambrosioides L. (Chenopodiaceae)	Curacao; South Carolina, U.S.; widely used in other warm countries	Plant infusion (or fresh juice) as a vermifuge, diuretic, sudorific, antispasmodic, etc; popular herb tea in France, Bolivia, Mexico	Terpenes	Tumors at injection site in 53% of rats, plant extract, s.c. dosing (19).
Croton flavens L. (Euphorbiaceae)	Curacao, Coro	Leafy branch tip decoction as a beverage, tonic for colds, stomach ache, rheumatism, etc.	Alkaloids, phorbol ester irritants	Irritant factor co-carcinogenic on the back skin of mice (40).
Diospyros virginiana L. (Ebenaceae)	South Carolina	Leaf decoction as beverage; dried unripe fruit infusion in chronic dysentery, uterine hemorrhage, sore throat gargle	Tannin	Tumors at injection site in 57% of rats, leaf extract, s.c. dosing (19).
Heliotropium ternatum Vahl (Boraginaceae)	Curacao	Plant decoction for menstrual cramps, leukorrhea; as diuretic, emmenagogue	—	Esophageal papillomas in 11% of hamsters, pulverized plant in cheek pouch (39).
Krameria ixina L. (Krameriaceae)	Curacao, Coro, Brazil	Plant decoction as tonic for liver, kidneys; emmenagogue, abortifacient, astringent in diarrhea, dysentery	Tannin	Fibrocarcinomas at injection site in 100% of rats, plant extract, s.c. dosing. No tumors with a tannin-free extract (37, 41). Multiple small papillomas in esophagus in 25% of hamsters, pulverized leaf stem with Ca(OH)₂.
Limonium nashii Small (Plumbaginaceae)	South Carolina	Root decoction for colds, fever, diarrhea; formerly as injection in gonorrhea, gleet, leukorrhea, prolapsus ani and uteri	Tannin	Tumors in 17% of rats, root extract, s.c. dosing (10).
Melochia tomentosa L. (Sterculiaceae)	Curacao, Coro	Root decoction for stomach ache, chronic diarrhea; as sore throat gargle, emmenagogue	Tannin, isatins, alkaloids, coumarins	Fibrocarcinoma at injection site in 100% of rats, root extract, s.c. dosing (37).
Myrica cerifera L. (Myricaceae)	South Carolina	Leaf tea as beverage, for back pain; leaf and twig decoction for diarrhea, severe colds, fever	Tannin, phenolics	Fibrocarcinoma at injection site in 27% of rats, tannin fraction from root extract, s.c. dosing; 33% with tannin-free phenolic fractions (10).
Quercus falcata var. *pagodaefolia* Ell. (Fagaceae)	South Carolina	Inner bark decoction for colds, fever, rheumatism, backache; to color whiskey	Tannin	Fibrocarcinoma at injection site in 100% of rats, bark extract, s.c. dosing; 93% with tannin fraction (10).
Rhus copallina L. (Anacardiaceae)	South Carolina	Root decoction in treating leukorrhea and gonorrhea	Tannin	Tumors at injection site in 33% of rats, root extract, s.c. dosing (19).
Sassafras albidum Nees (Lauraceae)	South Carolina	Root decoction as beverage, for fever, pneumonia, bronchitis, mumps	Safrole	Tumors at injection site in 67% of rats, root extract, s.c. dosing (19).

[a]   Detailed account of the plants and their use is given in References 24 and 36.

list a series of common plant names with no botanical names provided and no indication at all of the percentage of each included in the mixture. Some advertisements seem to imply that the more numerous the ingredients, the more magical the "health" benefits! Only a very few of the plant materials exploited as sources of "healthful, refreshing beverages" are properly classifiable as beverage plants. Outstanding among these few are leaves and stems of *Aspalathus linearis* (Burman filius) R. Dahlgren (Leguminosae); rooibos (or rooibosch) tea (or tee) from South Africa, and *Hibiscus sabdariffa* L. (Malvaceae), roselle, always mislabeled "hibiscus flowers," "hibiscus flores," or "flor de hibiscus."

Most of the plant materials sold in health food stores and by the natural-product dealers for beverage purposes were never meant to be so utilized. They are, in the main, oldtime medicinal plants long ago dropped from official practice in this country as either ineffective or harmful. Not only do many have physiologically active or toxic factors but they are packaged singly or in combinations with no warning of chemical properties and possible side-effects. Some of these so-called "beverages" are even being advocated for the relief of sundry ailments. But, as with all crude botanicals, there is no such thing as a measured dose because of the variability of the chemistry of the growing and harvested plant. Then, too, one cannot assume that the customer is invariably hale and hearty and unlikely to be affected by the active principles in a ''tea'' which he or she may imbibe nonchalantly several times a day every day of the week.

As discussed earlier, both epidemiological studies and bioassays in experimental animals suggest a strong correlation between the consumption of certain tannin-rich herbal teas and the incidence of esophageal cancer. A number of the obsolete medicinal plants currently marketed in health food stores as herbal teas for beverage use are noted for their tannin content in addition to possessing other active properties such as: (1) squaw tea, the dried branches of *Ephedra virdis* Cov. (Ephedraceae), (2) bayberry, *Myrica cerifera* L. (Myricaceae), (3) comfrey, *Symphytum officinale* L. (Boraginaceae), and (4) yellow dock tea, *Rumex crispus* L. (Polygonaceae). Among these, the tannin fractions from bayberry and comfrey have been found to be carcinogenic in rats.[10,31]

The antinutrient role of tannin is now being capitalized upon in the launching of a new product called ''Diet Partner''. Ingredients are listed as rose hips, blackberry leaves (high in tannin), hawthorne berries (also high in tannin), roasted chicory root, lemongrass, and ''hibiscus flowers,'' the latter two obviously for flavoring. The proportions of each are not stated, but the tannin-containing materials must make up a large part because of the implication in the tape-measure motif of the ''cover design'' and in the printed message: ''It can be drunk hot or cold as an accompaniment to your diet and exercise program. It is highly drinkable — suitable at any time of day and with meals, which is what makes it a dieter's partner.'' Tannin intake does, indeed, interfere with the body's utilization of protein; in cattle and chick feeds it shows a deficit in weight gain.[32,33] Anyone drinking high-tannin tea, conventional or herbal, even peppermint or spearmint which have appreciable tannin levels, and endeavoring to improve health by investing in high-protein bread and cereal would be treading a counterproductive pathway!

A list of herbal teas commonly sold in health food stores which pose carcinogenic hazard is given in Table 2. Available information on the carcinogenic activity of these teas in animal experiments is also included.

V. SUMMARY AND CONCLUSIONS

Like most things in life, overindulgence in any substance, even a particular component of normal diet, is clearly contraindicated. Available data on common tea suggest that its consumption in moderation may not have any significant ill effect on health. The potential risk may further be reduced by drinking tea with milk which appears to nullify the carcinogenic tannin through its protein binding action, at least in the upper digestive tract. The impact of tannin after it has been liberated from protein in the digestive process is not yet known. There is an indication that moderate tea consumption may have some specific health benefits such as anticarcinogenic effect due to its high fluoride content.[34] Also, other herbal teas may have some rewards[35] due to the presence of vitamins (e.g., vitamin C in rose hips), appetite stimulants (in chamomile) and gastric stimulants (in mint), but all of these favorable factors can be found in alternate beverages free of chemical carcinogens.

The recent epidemiological surveys provide persuasive data for possible correlations between excessive consumption of certain tannin-rich teas and the incidence of esophageal cancer. However, one has to be careful in interpreting such data since other possible contributing factors need to be thoroughly investigated. These may include lifestyle and the general health status of the particular population surveyed, and concurrent exposure to cocarcinogens or other known carcinogens such as tobacco (especially if chewed or taken as snuff), betel nut, red wine, dry cider, liquor aged in oak barrels or aged with oak chips, and high-phenol cultivars of sorghum, finger millet, or maize. While good leads have opened up, clearly there is a need for more research in firmly establishing the consumption of herbal teas as a cause of esophageal cancer in humans.

Table 2
HERBAL TEAS COMMONLY SOLD IN HEALTH FOOD STORES WHICH POSE CARCINOGENIC HAZARD

Common name(s)	Botanical name, species (family)	Plant part(s), use[a]	Chemical constituent(s) found to be carcinogenic in rats (references in parentheses)
Bayberry	*Myrica cerifera* L. (Myricaceae)	Leaves, flowers, bark; as beverage, for diarrhea, sore throat, colds, fever	Tannin and tannin-free phenolic fractions (10)
Calamus	*Acorus calamus* (Acraceae)	Rhizome; as aromatic, tonic, to flavor liquors	β-Asarone (45)
Coltsfoot, farfara	*Tussilago farfara* (Compositae)	Buds for cough	Senkirkine (46) and buds (47)
Comfrey	*Symphytum officinale* (Boraginaceae)	Leaves, roots, rhizome; as tonic, for ulcers	Symphytine and extracts of leaf and root (31)
Golden ragwort	*Senecio aureus* (Compositae)	Whole plant except roots; as emmenagogue	Senecionine (48)
Sassafras	*Sassafras albidum* Nees (Lauraceae)	Roots; as beverage, "blood thinner," for fever, pneumonia, etc.	Safrole (27) and safrole-free extract of roots (19)

[a] Detailed account of the plants and their use is given in References 35, 42 to 44.

The general public is largely unaware of the health risks involved in the indiscriminate and quantity consumption of herbal teas. This is due primarily to the erroneous stance promulgated by the health food stores that "if it is natural it is good," and that herbal teas are a safe means of avoiding caffeine. In addition to the occasional allergic reactions, there is a possibility that some constituents of herbal tea may adversely affect the therapeutic efficacy of vital medications by interfering with drug metabolism and bioavailability.

It is hoped that the scientists and health professionals will take the initiative in educating the public on the hazards involved in the casual and excessive drinking of herbal teas. There is an urgent need for the local, state, and federal regulatory agencies to assume jurisdiction through proper legal avenues and prevent the sale of clearly harmful and sometimes unsanitary herbal preparations by the health food stores and other "natural food" outlets.

Perhaps among the numerous herbal teas used around the world, there could well be substitutes that are appetizing and wholesome, and worthy of being widely promoted as alternatives to common tea and coffee. Study of such teas deserves the attention of the scientific community and the energy and resources of the beverage industry.

ACKNOWLEDGMENTS

Studies at Howard University were supported in part by contract Number N01 CP33266 from the National Cancer Institute and in part by the MBRS Grant Number 2 506RR-08016-11 from the National Institutes of Health and the National Cancer Institute.

REFERENCES

1. **Pfeiffer, C. J., Ed.,** *Cancer of the Esophagus,* Volumes 1 and 2, CRC Press, Boca Raton, Fla., 1982.
2. **Klassen, K. P.,** Dilemma of esophageal cancer, *JAMA,* 235, 1044, 1976.
3. **Anon.,** On the track of oesophageal cancer, *Food Cosmet. Toxicol.,* 19, 781, 1981.
4. **Anon.,** A world view of cancer, *Food Cosmet. Toxicol.,* 9, 897, 1971.
5. **Manakanit, W., Muir, C. S., and Jain, D. K.,** Cancer in Chiang Mai, North Thailand: a relative frequency study, *Br. J. Cancer,* 25, 225, 1971.
6. **Kumar, K. M. and Ramachandran, P.,** Carcinoma of oesophagus in Kerala, *Indian J. Cancer,* 10, 183, 1973.
7. **Segi, M.,** Tea-gruel as a possible factor for cancer of the esophagus, *Gann,* 66, 199, 1975.

8. Joint Iran-International Agency for Research on Cancer Study Group, Esophageal cancer studies in the Caspian littoral of Iran: results of population studies — a prodrome, *J. Natl. Cancer Inst.*, 59, 1127, 1977.
9. **Shimizu, T., Ueshima, I., and Masuda, C.,** A ten-year follow-up study of the relationship between tea gruel and gastric cancer, *Nippon Koshu Eisel Zasshi*, 27, 237, 1980.
10. **Kapadia, G. J., Paul, B. D., Chung, E. B., Ghosh, B., and Pradhan, S. N.,** Carcinogenicity of *Camellia sinensis* (Tea) and some tannin-containing folk medicinal herbs administered subcutaneously in rats, *J. Natl. Cancer Inst.*, 57, 207, 1976.
11. **Harlar, C. R.,** *Tea Manufacture,* Oxford University Press, Oxford, 1963, 126.
12. **Morton, J. F.,** Further association of plant tannins and human cancer, *Q. J. Crude Drug Res.*, 12, 1829, 1972.
13. **Miles, R. W.,** personal communication, 1975.
14. **Morton, J. F.,** Search for carcinogenic principles, in *Recent Advances in Phytochemistry, Vol. 14, The Resource Potential in Phytochemistry,* Swain, T. and Kleiman, R., Eds., Plenum Press, New York, 1980, 61.
15. **Kaiser, H. E. and Bartone, J. C.,** The carcinogenic activity of ordinary tea: a preliminary note, *J. Natl. Med. Assoc.*, 58, 361, 1966.
16. **Kaiser, H. E.,** Cancer-promoting effects of phenols in tea, *Cancer*, 10, 614, 1967.
17. **Raghavan, V. and Baruah, H. K.,** Arecanut: India's popular masticatory — history, chemistry and utilization, *Econ. Bot.*, 12, 315, 1958.
18. **Dunham, L. J.,** A geographic study of the relationship between oral cancer and plants, *Cancer Res.*, 28, 2369, 1968.
19. **Kapadia, G. J., Chung, E. B., Ghosh, B., Shukla, Y. N., Basak, S. P., Morton, J. F., and Pradhan, S. N.,** Carcinogenicity of some folk medicinal herbs in rats, *J. Natl. Cancer Inst.*, 60, 683, 1978.
20. **Ranadive, K. J., Ranadive, S. N., Shivapurkar, N. M., and Gothoskar, S. V.,** Betel quid chewing and oral cancer: experimental studies on hamsters, *Int. J. Cancer*, 24, 835, 1977.
21. **Gendorn, Y., Ardouin, C., Lassale, Y., and Sirol, J.,** Cancer of the esophagus in Djibouti. Report of 36 cases collected in two years, *Bull. Soc. Pathol. Exp.*, 70, 74, 1977.
22. **Getahun, A. and Krikorian, A. D.,** Chat: coffee's rival from Harar, Ethiopia. I. Botany, cultivation and use, *Econ. Bot.*, 27, 353, 1973.
23. **Prudente, A.,** Patologia geografica do cancer no Brasil, *Boletim Oncologia*, 46, 281, 1963.
24. **Morton, J. F.,** *Folk Remedies of the Low Country,* Seeman Publishing, Miami, Fla., 1974, 176.
25. **Bär, S. and Griepentrog, F.,** Die Situation in der gesundheitlischen Beurteilung der Aromatisie für Lebensmittel, *Med. Ernaehr.*, 8, 244, 1967.
26. **Grieve, M.,** *A Modern Herbal,* Hafner Press, New York, 1967, 888.
27. **Long, E. L., Nelson, A. A., Fitzhugh, O. G., and Hansen, W. H.,** Liver tumors produc feeding safrole, *Arch. Pathol.*, 75, 595, 1963.
28. **Long, E. L. and Jenner, P. M.,** Esophageal tumors produced in rats by the feeding of di *Fed. Proc. Fed. Am. Soc. Exp. Biol.*, 22, 275, 1963.
29. **Koike, K., Ogura, M., and Farnsworth, N. R.,** Personal communication, 1976.
30. **Morton, J. F.,** Tentative correlations of plant usage and esophageal cancer zones, *Econ. B* 1970.
31. **Hirono, I., Mori, H., and Haga, M.,** Carcinogenic activity of *Symphytum officinale, J. N Inst.*, 61, 865, 1978.
32. **Bertrand, J. E. and Lutrick, M. C.,** The feeding value of bird-resistant and non-bird-resistan grain in the ration of beef steers, *Sunshine State Agric. Res. Rep.*, 16, 16, 1971.
33. **Price, M. L., Butler, L. G., Rogler, J. C., and Featherston, W. R.,** Overcoming the nutrit harmful effects of tannin in sorghum grain by treatment with inexpensive chemicals, *J. Agric. Food Chem.*, 27, 441, 1979.
34. **Rosen, S. and Elvin-Lewis, M.,** Anticarcinogenic effect of tea in rats, *J. Dent. Res.*, 61, 326, 1982.
35. **Lewis, H. W. and Elvin-Lewis, M. P. F.,** *Medical Botany: Plants Affecting Man's Health,* J. Wiley & Sons, New York, 1977, 388.
36. **Morton, J. F.,** *Atlas of Medicinal Plants of Middle America,* Charles C Thomas, Springfield, Ill., 1981.
37. **O'Gara, R. W., Lee, C. W., Morton, J. F., Kapadia, G. J., and Dunham, L. J.,** Sarcoma in rats from extracts of whole plants and from fractionated extracts of *Krameria ixina, J. Natl. Cancer Inst.*, 52, 445, 1974.
38. **Pradhan, S. N., Chung, E. B., Ghosh, B., Paul, B. D., and Kapadia, G. J.,** Potential carcinogens. I. Carcinogenicity of some plant extracts and their tannin-containing fractions in rats, *J. Natl. Cancer Inst.*, 52, 1579, 1974.
39. **Dunham, L. J., Sheets, R. H., and Morton, J. F.,** Proliferative lesions in cheek pouch and esophagus of hamsters treated with plants from Curacao, Netherlands Antilles, *J. Natl. Cancer Inst.*, 53, 1259, 1974.
40. **Weber, J. and Hecker, E.,** Carcinogens of the diterpene ester type from *Croton flavens* L. and esophageal cancer in Curacao, *Experientia*, 34, 679, 1978.

41. **O'Gara, R. W., Lee, C., and Morton, J. F.,** Carcinogenicity of extracts of selected plants from Curacao after oral and subcutaneous administration to rodents, *J. Natl. Cancer Inst.,* 46, 1131, 1971.
42. **Morton, J. F.,** Is there a safer tea? *Morris Arbor. Bull.,* 26, 24, 1975.
43. **Der Marderosian, A.,** Medicinal teas - boon or bane? *Drug Ther.,* 7(2), 178, 1977.
44. **Tyler, V. E., Brady, L. R., and Robbers, J. E.,** Herbs and "Health Foods," *Pharmacognosy,* 8th ed., Lea & Febiger, Philadelphia, 1981, 468.
45. **Taylor, J. M., Jones, W. I., Hagan, E. C., Gross, M. A., Davis, D. A., and Cook, E. L.,** Toxicity of oil of calamus (Jammu variety), *Toxicol. Appl. Pharmacol.,* 10, 405, 1967.
46. **Hirono, I., Haga, M., Fuji, M., Matsuura, S., Matsubara, M., Nakayama, M., Furuya, T., Hikichi, M., Takanashi, H., Uchida, E., Hosaka, S., and Ueno, I.,** Induction of hepatic tumors in rats by senkirkine and symphytine, *J. Natl. Cancer Inst.,* 63, 469, 1979.
47. **Hirono, I., Mori, H., and Culvenor, C. C. J.,** Carcinogenic activity of coltsfoot, *Tussilago farfara* L., *Gann,* 67, 125, 1976.
48. **Cook, J. W., Duffy, E., and Schoental, R.,** Primary liver tumors in rats following feeding with alkaloids of *Senecio jacobaea, Br. J. Cancer,* 4, 405, 1950.

Chapter 2

COFFEE AND CANCER

A. B. Miller

TABLE OF CONTENTS

I. INTRODUCTION

Coffee is a widely used natural product mainly consumed as a beverage but used also as a flavoring in manufactured foods, though the latter usage has been largely replaced by synthetic products.

The possibility that coffee consumption may increase the risk of cancer in man was first raised in relation to bladder cancer and more recently in relation to pancreatic cancer. Not unnaturally, this has excited wide public interest, especially in relation to pancreatic cancer, though this interest was somewhat short-lived and the sensational news reports that accompanied the release of one of the articles concerning the association resulted also in considerable public skepticism.

It is not the purpose of this review to consider the implications of such publicity on cancer control generally, but the author shall consider the difficulties in determining whether associations of this type demonstrated by epidemiologic studies are causal. Further, it is not the author's intent to discuss animal experimental data, but in considering this review of epidemiologic studies it is appropriate to keep in the back of one's mind that Hueper and others[1] produced data that suggested that the soot of coffee-roasting plants may be carcinogenic, and identified carcinogenic hydrocarbons in roasted coffee.[2] Nevertheless, long-term feeding studies in rats conducted by General Foods did not indicate any carcinogenic effect of instant coffee.[3]

II. BLADDER CANCER

Cole[4] conducted a population-based case control study on patients having cancer of the lower urinary tract and controls drawn from the same population. An unanticipated finding was an association of the disease with coffee drinking. The relative risk for coffee drinkers compared to non-drinkers was 1.24 among men and 2.58 among women. The association was strong in the sex-age groups in which associations of the disease with cigarette smoking and occupation are not strong. Cole pointed out that in an earlier case control study carried out in New Orleans,[5] an association between bladder cancer and coffee drinking was found which was not statistically significant overall. Subsequently, Fraumeni, Scotto, and Dunham[6] reanalyzed the data from this study using Cole's approach and found a significantly higher risk for black women who drank two or less cups of coffee per day. White women showed an opposite trend; white men and black men showed some evidence of increased risk, but no suggestion of a dose-response relationship. The inconsistency by race and sex and the lack of a dose-response relationship suggested to the author that the association may be indirect or non-causal. However, they did note a similar pattern when the analysis was limited to persons who never smoked. Bross and Tidings[7] reevaluated their own data and reported a weak positive association for men and a weak inverse one for women. Morgan and Jain,[8] in a case control study based on a mail questionnaire, found no evidence of increased risk for consumption of tea or coffee. Simon, Yen, and Cole,[9] in a case control study of white women with lower urinary tract cancer (again collecting data by a mail questionnaire), found an increased risk of bladder cancer for women who drank one or more cups of coffee a day (relative risk for 1 + cup/day coffee drinkers compared to none: 2.1). No dose-response relationship was demonstrated with usual daily coffee consumption or cups per years of coffee drinking nor did they find any differences in the association whether decaffeinated, nondecaffeinated regular, or instant coffee had been drunk. However, they found the highest risk (relative risk: 3.7) in those who were also moderate to heavy smokers. Wynder and Goldsmith[10] found positive associations for coffee drinking and bladder cancer in both men and women, with a dose-response relationship in men; the relative risk at highest coffee consumption levels for men is 2.0 after controlling for cigarette consumption. Morrison[11] evaluated bladder cancer incidence rates internationally in relation to per capita coffee imports for 10 countries and analyzed time trends for these variables for the U.S. and Denmark. Among the 10 countries there was a weak positive association between coffee and bladder cancer for both men and women. There was also a weak positive correlation of the time trends of coffee imports and bladder cancer incidence for men but not women in the U.S., however, in Denmark, the trends of coffee imports were dissimilar to both male and female trends in bladder cancer incidence. Morrison concluded that these results provided little support for an association of coffee drinking with the development of bladder cancer.

Mettlin and Graham,[12] in a study of dietary risk factors in bladder cancer, found some elevation of risk for heavy coffee drinking but again no particular evidence of a dose-response relationship. Howe et al.,[13] in a detailed study primarily initiated to evaluate coffee consumption, found an indication of increased risk in males for consumption of all types of coffee, regular coffee, and instant coffee and a slight but insignificant increase in risk for females (Table 1). However, it was found that there was an interaction between smoking and coffee drinking in females with an apparently significant increased risk for females who consumed both instant coffee and were cigarette smokers (Table 2). Although the increased risk in males persisted in logistic regression models controlling for cigarette use and other variables, there was no evidence of any increase in risk within increasing consumptions patterns of all types of coffee, of regular, or instant coffee. There was also no evidence of any increase in risk for consumption of tea in this or any other of the studies reporting on tea consumption, suggesting that if coffee consumption increases the risk of cancer, it is not because of caffeine intake. These findings were thus similar to those of Simon, Yen, and Cole.[9]

Cartwright et al.[14] found some increase in risk for male drinkers of instant coffee (relative risk = 1.5) but not for females. However, adjustment for cigarette smoking reduced the risk in men to insignificant levels (relative risk = 1.2).

Morrison et al.,[15] in a study conducted in Boston, Manchester, England, and Nagoya, Japan of a broadly based series of cases of lower urinary tract cancer and population controls, specifically evaluated the relationship with coffee drinking in these three areas. There was no evidence in any of the areas of increased risk with consumption of one or more cups of coffee per day even at consumption levels of five or six cups per day, with no evidence of a dose-response relationship. The authors concluded that apparent associations of coffee drinking and bladder cancer reported in the past may have been due to incomplete control of cigarette smoking. Although this conclusion may be valid it is of interest that in the study of Howe et al.[13] there was no evidence of any modification of the risk ratios by control of cigarette smoking, while in the earlier study of Cole[4] there was a suggestion that the coffee drinking effect might be particularly noted in those groups where there was little effect of smoking and occupational risk. However, the inconsistent findings in a number of studies and the absence of a dose-response relationship even when increased risk is demonstrated combine to suggest that the association when noted is not causal. Further clarification may be obtained by a second large case control study in Canada still in progress. Evidence may also be derived from the large U.S. study of bladder cancer risk on which so far only artificial sweetener consumption has been reported.[16]

III. PANCREATIC CANCER

A significant relationship between coffee consumption and pancreatic cancer mortality was reported by Stocks[17] a little over a decade ago among males in 20 countries. It is notable that the same study did not find an association between coffee consumption and bladder cancer. Lyon et al.[18] noted that non-Mormons in Utah have higher incidence rates of pancreatic cancer than Mormons, who consume less alcohol, tea, and coffee than non-Mormons.

Table 1
RELATIVE RISK ESTIMATES FOR CONSUMPTION OF COFFEE[13]

Type of coffee consumption	Males		Females	
	Discordant pairs[a]	Relative risk (95% confidence limits)	Discordant pairs[a]	Relative risk (95% confidence limits)
All types of coffee	66/48	1.4 (0.9—2.0)	20/19	1.0 (0.5—2.1)
Regular coffee	66/45	1.5 (1.0—2.2)	17/20	0.8 (0.4—1.7)
Instant coffee	116/79	1.5 (1.1—2.0)	30/21	1.4 (0.8—2.6)

[a]   No. of pairs: case ever used, control never used/case never used, control ever used.

Table 2
CASE-CONTROL DISTRIBUTION AND RELATIVE RISKS FOR INSTANT COFFEE CONSUMPTION BY SMOKING[13]

Smoking and coffee drinking status[a]	Number of		Relative risk	95% confidence limits
	Cases	Controls		
S − C −	71	96	1.0	
S + C −	55	47	1.6	0.9—2.7
S − C +	8	8	1.4	0.4—4.4
S + C +	18	1	24.3	3.3—501.0

[a]   S −: non-smokers; C −: average frequency coffee consumption less than 2 cups per day; S +: smoker; C +: average frequency coffee consumption more than 2 cups per day.

Subsequently, an association between coffee consumption and pancreatic cancer has been reported in two case control studies. Kessler and Lin[19] conducted a study of pancreatic cancer in over 115 hospitals in 5 metropolitan areas of the U.S. with hospital controls similar in age, sex, race, and marital status selected at random from among contemporaneous admissions to the same hospital. Interviews were conducted between 1972 and 1975 and 109 case control pairs were included in the analyses. The cases tended to drink more decaffeinated coffee than the controls. The difference was statistically significant for de-caffeinated coffee drinking among females. MacMahon et al.[20] questioned 369 patients with histologically proved cancer of the pancreas and 644 hospital controls; 273 had cancer other than cancers of the pancreas, biliary tract, respiratory tract, or bladder and 371 had other non-malignant disorders. A strong association between coffee consumption and pancreatic cancer was evident in both sexes which was not affected by controlling for cigarette smoking. There was some evidence of a dose-response relationship in females but not in males. No data were presented according to different types of coffee and the question on coffee was limited to the number of cups consumed in a typical day before the current illness was evident. The authors commented that in spite of the report of Kessler and Lin,[19] it seemed unlikely that decaffeinated coffee has a causal relation to pancreatic cancer in view of its relatively recent use. They felt it more likely that the high consumption of decaffeinated coffee noted by Kessler and Lin[19] was a reflection of generally high coffee consumption by patients in the past. MacMahon et al.[20] discussed the possibility that use of hospital controls resulted in a spurious increase in risk as such controls might have reduced their coffee consumption because of their illness. Indeed, Rosenberg et al.[21] noted a lower proportion of coffee consumers among hospitalized women with chronic disease than among women admitted with acute emergencies. However, MacMahon et al.[20] commented that the difference noted by Rosenberg et al.[21] was less than they had noted in their own study and that pancreatic cancer, being a chronic disease, would seem as likely as any other disorder to induce a change in coffee consumption.

One further aspect of the MacMahon et al.[20] study should be noted. Very few variables were analyzed and presumably other dietary variables that might be causally associated with pancreatic cancer were not ascertained, e.g., total fat consumption. Yet in international correlation studies of cancer incidence and dietary variables, a strong intercorrelation of total fat and coffee consumption has been noted (e.g., $r = 0.53$ in a study of Armstrong and Doll[22]). It is thus important not only that the association noted by MacMahon et al.[20] be further evaluated, but that such an evaluation include a detailed and preferably quantitative assessment of other, possibly more relevant, dietary variables.

It seems clear that a causal association between coffee drinking and pancreatic cancer has not yet been established though it seems very likely that a number of studies further evaluating the association will be conducted over the next few years.

IV. OTHER CANCERS

Other reported associations of coffee drinking with cancer have been scattered and inconsistent. Martinez[23] found an association between oral and esophageal cancers combined with consumption of hot beverages, said to be mostly coffee; Stocks[17] however, did not find a significant correlation between coffee consumption and esophageal cancer. Shennan[24] reported a positive correlation between per capita coffee consumption and mortality from renal carcinoma ($r = 0.8$), and the association, though less strong, was also found in the large study of Armstrong and Doll[22] correlating many environmental variables with cancer incidence and mortality. On the other hand, case-control studies of renal cancer[25,26] have not confirmed this association. Takahashi[27] and Stocks[17] found a positive correlation of prostate cancer mortality with per capita coffee consumption; this finding also appeared in the analysis by Armstrong and Doll[22] who reported a stronger association with total fat consumption and a high intercorrelation between these two dietary factors. However, prostate cancer incidence showed a stronger correlation with coffee consumption than total fat in this study. Other sites where Armstrong and Doll[22] showed a positive correlation between coffee consumption and cancer incidence or mortality were breast, corpus uteri, ovary, testis, kidney, and nervous system cancer. However, in each instance the correlation was higher with total fat consumption and often animal protein consumption and it seems probable that the findings for coffee were a reflection of intercorrelation between dietary variables.

V. METHODOLOGIC ISSUES

It is perhaps no accident that the studies that have reported positive associations between either bladder or pancreatic cancer and coffee consumption have been conducted by the case-control approach. A number of biases can affect case-control studies[28] and no one study can necessarily be free of all of them. However, for a risk factor (even if weak) to show an effect, generally one can expect consistency between studies, which providing they are conducted by different mechanisms would help to reassure one that the associations were not due to a systematic error present in all studies.

More difficult are the problems associated with elucidating information on exposure, particularly exposure very far in the past. Coffee consumption is perhaps particularly likely to be influenced by the occurrence of disease and indeed there have already been well documented circumstances in which admission to hospital for disease appears to have affected the consumption of coffee.[21] Considerable concern therefore arises over studies in which only current coffee consumption or very recent coffee consumption is ascertained. Fortunately, perhaps, coffee is not generally associated in the public consciousness with the occurrence of disease. Thus, although there may be difficulties in recall of consumption of coffee at periods in the lifetime which might be expected to be etiologically relevant for a cancer, such difficulties are likely to be equally represented among cases and controls so that recall bias may not be a problem. Nevertheless, changes of coffee consumption with disease make it necessary to be particularly cautious over the interpretation of studies in which hospital controls are used. It was a feature of the studies of bladder cancer and coffee that the initial observation arose in a study in which population controls were used and that the inconsistency which is present now arises over circumstances in which population controls have produced conflicting findings. However, for pancreatic cancer the only data currently available relates to hospital-based case-control studies.

In addition to the necessity to recall consumption in the past it is desirable that adequate information be obtained on the types of coffee consumed. However, even this requirement may be difficult to comply with in practice. Thus, Howe et al.,[13] in discussing somewhat different findings in males and females of coffee consumption and risk of bladder cancer suggest that males may be less knowledgeable than females about the type of coffee they consume; conceivably male consumers of instant coffee may believe that they are drinking regular coffee. This observation arose from the experience of the present author when he was included in a validation study for a dietary questionnaire in which it became clear that he had not appreciated that the coffee he consumed at mid-morning was instant coffee. This error raises the desirability that in case-control studies in which different types of coffee consumption are to be ascertained, the accuracy of the distinctions made should be confirmed possibly through spouse interviews.[13] Unfortunately at times it is difficult to obtain confirmation on types of coffee consumed even from spouses, especially regarding consumption in the distant past.

Even if accuracy over type of coffee can be assumed it is still necessary to decide how coffee consumption will be categorized in an analysis. As current coffee consumption seems least likely to be relevant some attempt has to be made to quantify the amount of coffee that individuals have consumed in the past. In our first attempts to analyze the data from our study of bladder cancer we developed cumulative measures of consumption, possible because we obtained information both on frequency and duration of consumption for every period in the lifetime of cases or controls when this frequency differed.[29] In the definitive analyses[13] we considered current consumption, average (lifetime) frequency, and total lifetime consumption. The results obtained were generally similar, particularly for average frequency and total lifetime consumption. As both these measures seem theoretically preferable to current consumption and as average frequency seems more interpretable than cumulative numbers of cups consumed in a lifetime, we presented our results in terms of average frequency as cups per day.

If coffee consumption is causal for bladder cancer it is clearly a relatively weak cause, though because of its ubiquity, our own calculations would suggest a population attributable risk of 21% in males and 12% in females.[13] If, as our results suggest, it is particularly likely to increase risk in association with cigarette consumption in women, and if it acts as a promoter, a dose-response relationship is not necessarily going to be demonstrable. Part of the difficulty in unravelling any causal association, as pointed out by Morrison et al.,[15] is the tendency for consumers of coffee to be also heavy users of cigarettes. In spite of sophisticated techniques of analysis, unless there are sufficient individuals who do not smoke yet consume substantial amounts of coffee it will be extremely difficult to demonstrate significant associations. Somewhat surprisingly Morrison et al.[15] presented their findings in terms of current consumption. However, the uniformly negative findings in a study of populations which differ in their coffee consumption do cast substantial doubt on the causality of the association in other studies.

Feinstein et al.[30] have published a critical commentary on the MacMahon et al.[20] case-control study of pancreatic cancer. They point out that if, as a result of some of the errors and biases inseparable from a hospital-based case-control study, there had been relatively minor amounts of misclassification of pancreatic cancer cases who were noncoffee drinkers as coffee drinkers and controls who were coffee drinkers as noncoffee drinkers, then the reported association could vanish. They also comment on the number of contrasts that were evaluated and the necessity to modify statistical significance levels under these circumstances. Their criticisms seem a little harsh and in particular, it is difficult to accept that pancreatic cancer cases who were truly noncoffee drinkers would be misclassified as coffee drinkers. Nevertheless, further studies of the association in which lifetime histories of coffee consumption are obtained, in which population based series of cases and population based series of controls are also ascertained, and adequate evaluation conducted for interaction with other causal factors in the diet are badly needed. However, it should be noted that one of the difficulties Feinstein et al.[30] comment on, namely that many of the cancer cases that were ascertained were not interviewed because they had died, will always be a difficulty in case-control studies of rapidly progressive fatal cancers such as pancreatic cancer. The absence of cases of such a type from case-control studies means that one has to be careful in assessing results and that it should not be assumed that findings derived from series which do not include rapidly progressive cases necessarily apply to the total universe of cases.

In conclusion, the lack of consistency in the findings in a number of different case-control studies and the absence of a dose-response relationship even in those studies which showed an association suggests that the reported associations between coffee consumption and bladder cancer are non-causal. For pancreatic cancer the stronger risk levels found in one study, the presence of a dose-response relationship in females, and the finding of associations internationally between mortality from pancreatic cancer and coffee consumption suggests that the association could eventually turn out to be causal, though before such a conclusion is justified further studies must be conducted that include appropriate consideration of other dietary variables, especially total fat consumption. Thus further work is undoubtedly required and it may be some years before definitive conclusions are possible. In the meantime it is hoped that any study in which data on coffee consumption was obtained in a group of individuals who have been kept under observation for a period and in whom the incidence of pancreatic and bladder cancer can be ascertained should be fully analyzed as it is possible that only the cohort approach will provide the definitive answers required to the questions that have been posed by the case-control studies so far reported.

REFERENCES

1. **Hueper, W. C. and Payne, W. W.,** Carcinogenic studies on soot of coffee-roasting plants, *AMA Arch. Pathol.,* 69, 716, 1960.
2. **Kuratsune, M. and Hueper, W. C.,** Polycyclic aromatic hydrocarbons in roasted coffee, *J. Natl. Cancer Inst.,* 24, 463, 1960.
3. **Zeitlin, B. R.,** Coffee and bladder cancer, *Lancet,* 1, 1066, 1972.
4. **Cole, P.,** Coffee-drinking and cancer of the lower urinary tract, *Lancet,* 1, 1335, 1971.
5. **Dunham, L. J., Rabson, A. S., Stewart, H. L., Frank, A. S., and Young, J. L., Jr.,** Rates, interview, and pathology study of cancer of the urinary bladder in New Orleans, Louisiana, *J. Natl. Cancer Inst.,* 41, 683, 1968.
6. **Fraumeni, J. F., Jr., Scotto, J., and Dunham, L. J.,** Coffee-drinking and bladder cancer, *Lancet,* 2, 1204, 1971.
7. **Bross, I. D. and Tidings, J.,** Another look at coffee-drinking and cancer of the urinary bladder, *Prev. Med.,* 2, 445, 1973.

8. **Morgan, R. W. and Jain, M. G.,** Bladder cancer: smoking, beverages and artificial sweeteners, *Can. Med. Assoc. J.,* 111, 1067, 1974.
9. **Simon, D., Yen, S., and Cole, P.,** Coffee drinking and cancer of the lower urinary tract, *J. Natl. Cancer Inst.,* 54, 587, 1975.
10. **Wynder, E. L. and Goldsmith, R.,** The epidemiology of bladder cancer — a second look, *Cancer,* 40, 1246, 1977.
11. **Morrison, A. S.,** Geographic and time trends of coffee imports and bladder cancer, *Eur. J. Cancer,* 14, 51, 1978.
12. **Mettlin, C. and Graham, S.,** Dietary risk factors in human bladder cancer, *Am. J. Epidemiol.,* 110, 255, 1979.
13. **Howe, G. R., Burch, J. D., Miller, A. B., Cook, G. M., Esteve, J., Morrison, B., Gordon, P., Chambers, L. W., Fodor, G., and Winsor, G. M.,** Tobacco use, occupation, coffee, various nutrients and bladder cancer, *J. Natl. Cancer Inst.,* 64, 701, 1980.
14. **Cartwright, R. A., Adib, R., Glashan, R., and Gray, B. K.,** The epidemiology of bladder cancer in West Yorkshire. A preliminary report on non-occupational aetiologies, *Carcinogenesis,* 2, 343, 1981.
15. **Morrison, A. S., Buring, J. E., Verhoek, W. G., Aoki, K., Leck, I., Ohno, Y., and Obata, K.,** Coffee drinking and cancer of the lower urinary tract, *J. Natl. Cancer Inst.,* 68, 91, 1982.
16. **Hoover, R. N. and Strasser, P. H.,** Artificial sweeteners and human bladder cancer. Preliminary results, *Lancet,* 302, 837, 1980.
17. **Stocks, P..** Cancer mortality in relation to national consumption of cigarettes, solid fuel, tea and coffee, *Br. J. Cancer,* 24, 215, 1970.
18. **Lyon, J. L., Gardner, J. W., and West, D. W.** Cancer risk and life-style: cancer among Mormons from 1967—1975, in *Cancer Incidence in Defined Populations,* Banbury Report No. 4, Cairns, J., Lyon, J. L., and Skolnick, M., Eds., Cold Spring Harbor Laboratory, Cold Spring Harbor, N.Y., 1980, 3.
19. **Kessler, I. I. and Lin, R. S.,** A multifactorial model for pancreatic cancer in man, *JAMA,* 245, 147, 1981.
20. **MacMahon, B., Yen, S., Trichopoulos, D., Warren, K., and Nardi, G.,** Coffee and cancer of the pancreas, *New Engl. J. Med.,* 304, 630, 1981.
21. **Rosenberg, L., Slone, D., Shapiro, S., Kaufman, D. W., Stolley, P. D., and Miettinen, O. S.,** Coffee drinking and myocardial infection in young women, *Am. J. Epidemiol.,* 111, 675, 1980.
22. **Armstrong, B. and Doll, R.,** Environmental factors and cancer incidence and mortality in different countries, with special reference to dietary practices, *Int. J. Cancer,* 15, 617, 1975.
23. **Martinez, I.,** Factors associated with cancer of the esophagus, mouth and pharynx in Puerto Rico, *J. Natl. Cancer Inst.,* 42, 1069, 1969.
24. **Shennan, D. H.,** Renal carcinoma and coffee consumption in 16 countries, *Br. J. Cancer,* 28, 473, 1973.
25. **Wynder, E. L., Mabuchi, K., and Whitmore, W. F.,** Epidemiology of adenocarcinoma of the kidney, *J. Natl. Cancer Inst.,* 53, 1619, 1974.
26. **Armstrong, B., Garrod, A., and Doll, R.,** A retrospective study of renal cancer with special reference to coffee and animal protein consumption, *Br. J. Cancer,* 33, 127, 1976.
27. **Takahashi, E.,** Coffee consumption and mortality for prostate cancer, *Tohoku J. Exp. Med.,* 82, 218, 1964.
28. **Sackett, D. L.,** Bias in analytic research, *J. Chron. Dis.,* 32, 51, 1979.
29. **Miller, A. B.,** The etiology of bladder cancer from the epidemiologic viewpoint, *Cancer Res.,* 37, 2939, 1977.
30. **Feinstein, A. R., Horwitz, R. I., Spitzer, W. O., and Battista, R. N.,** Coffee and pancreatic cancer. The problems of etiologic science and epidemiologic case-control research, *JAMA,* 246, 957, 1981.

Chapter 3

SALTED FISH AND NASOPHARYNGEAL CARCINOMA

Dolly P. Huang and J. H. C. Ho

TABLE OF CONTENTS

I. INTRODUCTION

The predominant malignant neoplasm arising in the nasopharynx of people of different races is a carcinoma of the squamous type. It frequently appears under light microscopy in the poorly differentiated or undifferentiated forms, but under electron microscopy, features of squamous differentiation, e.g., desmosomes and tonofilaments, could be identified in the apparently undifferentiated tumor.[1] Lymphoepithelioma and transitional cell carcinoma are no longer considered as separate pathological entities but simply as variants of squamous carcinoma, and it is in this type of nasopharyngeal carcinoma (NPC) that salted fish consumption has been suspected to be a risk factor. The suspicion was first raised by Ho[2] because salted fish has been traditionally a very popular food item among southern, but not northern, Chinese, in and outside China, in Macaonese of mixed Portuguese and Chinese ancestry, and Malaysians, and these people have a high risk for cancer.

In this chapter we attempt to summarize and review the epidemiological and experimental evidence related to the hypothesis.

II. EPIDEMIOLOGICAL EVIDENCE

NPC has been known to be prevalent among southern Chinese in Canton as early as 1921[3] and in Singapore even as early as 1912.[4] It is, therefore, likely that the major environmental risk factor, if one was involved, was associated with the traditional rather than modern lifestyle of southern Chinese, and that it was one that southern Chinese brought along with them when they migrated to distant lands. The question is whether the major factor is an ingestant or inhalant.

First, Dobson[5] postulated that NPC in Chinese was caused by frequent and prolonged exposures to the smoke from burning grass, wood, tobacco, candles, incense (joss sticks), kerosene lamps, and lamps burning peanut oil in poorly ventilated houses in China. Later, his smoke inhalation hypothesis received support from observations by workers in Kenya.[6,7] The evidence was reviewed by Ho[8,9] who argued against the hypothesis, basing his arguments on the following observations:

1. A male preponderance for the disease when it is the females who are more exposed to household smoke.
2. People who lived in boats and cook in the open in Hong Kong have an incidence rate significantly higher than the land-dwellers living in crowded quarters.[10]
3. Southern Chinese living in well-ventilated dwellings in Hong Kong and Singapore have no less risk of developing NPC than their rural countrymen in China.
4. NPC was rare among the large number of Buddhist monks in Hangzhou before the last war and they spent much of their time in an incense-laden atmosphere.[11] However, the cancer was not rare in Catholic Macaonese and Muslim Malays, neither of whom burn Chinese incense.

In favor of the ingestant hypothesis is the observation that Chinese who have settled overseas tend to retain much of their food culture and this applies particularly to the consumption of salted fish.[9,12] Furthermore, the boat-dwelling fisherfolks who have the highest risk for NPC tend to consume salted fish more frequently than land-dwelling Chinese in Hong Kong. A study of the age-specific incidence curves of NPC in Hong Kong, where over 98% of the population were classified as Chinese and of predominantly southern origin by successive censuses in 1961, 1971, and 1981, showed that the initiation of the carcinogenesis occurred most probably during early childhood.[12-14] It has been revealed in a study on the cultural and social factors relating to Chinese infant feeding and weaning that among the traditional foods frequently fed to southern Chinese in the weaning and post-weaning period is salted fish added to congee, a rice porridge.[15] A retrospective study of the early environmental backgrounds of young Chinese NPC patients found that salted fish was among the traditional foods most commonly eaten by the patients and fed to them when they were babies.[16]

Another study, one of the socioeconomic status, past health and food habits of 150 NPC patients and 150 age- and sex-matched controls consisting of patients with other cancers hospitalized in Queen Elizabeth Hospital, Hong Kong, undertaken by a team of workers from the International Agency for Research on Cancer (IARC), collaborating with those in the Medical and Health Department Institute of Radiology and Oncology, disclosed that salted fish was given to babies just after weaning more often in households with an NPC patient than in control households. A multivariate analysis of the data collected from the study showed that traditional lifestyle and the consumption of salted fish during weaning were independent risk factors for NPC.[17]

Hirayama[18] studied the correlation between the age-adjusted incidence rate per 100,000 for NPC and the consumption of animal protein, fruits, and salted fish as indicated by the ratio of daily intake of salted fish to the daily intake of raw fish, and the number of Chinese per 100,000 in the population in 9 districts in Japan. He found a negative correlation between NPC incidence and animal protein or fruit consumption, but a relatively high positive correlation (correlation coefficient $r = 0.711$) for salted fish consumption, which was higher than that for the proportion of Chinese in the population ($r = 0.579$).

In an epidemiological study carried out in Alaska among natives consisting of Eskimos, Indians, and Aleuts, who have a risk for NPC intermediate between the risk for southern Chinese and that for Caucasians, the NPC patients in response to a questionnaire more often reported the use of salted fish in their childhood diet, but the difference was not significant.[19]

A study designed to further examine the role of inhaled carcinogens and the ingestion of salted fish as risk factors in NPC in Chinese in Hong Kong and Los Angeles by comparing their incidence rates, and by such factors as age, sex, birthplace, and occupation concluded that the incidence data coupled with available experimental evidence are most consistent with consumption of Cantonese salted fish as the major risk factor.[20]

A case-control survey among 100 Chinese NPC patients and 100 Chinese control participants matched to a case by sex, age group (within 5 years), and neighborhood of residence for at least 5 years in 27 census districts of the Klang Valley in the State of Selangor, Malaya, Malaysia[21] has just been completed. In this study no difference has been found between case and control participants in current eating of salted fish, but the pattern of consumption in childhood and in adolescence was highly significant. In childhood a strong dose-response relationship was revealed, and in adolescence a similar relationship, although weaker, is also apparent.

III. EXPERIMENTAL EVIDENCE

It is well-known that nitrosamines can induce malignant tumors in a wide variety of organs in many animal species, and several nitrosamines are known to induce squamous carcinomas, adenocarcinomas, and other tumors in the nasal and paranasal cavities or nasopharyngeal tube of experimental animals.[22-26] It has been shown that nitrosamines have an organotropic carcinogenic effect, causing carcinomas to develop in susceptible tissues irrespective of the route of their administration to the animal.[27] It is therefore logical to look for the presence of nitrosamines in salted fish as a first step. On the suggestion of Ho, Fong and Walsh[28] reported the finding of a high content of *N*-nitrosodimethylamine (NDMA) and *N*-nitroso-diethylamine (NDEA) at 0.6 to 9 ppm and 1.2 to 21 ppm, respectively in four species of salted, ungutted marine fish (anchovies, croakers, yellow croakers, and white herrings) using thin layer chromatography (TLC) following the method of Sen et al.[29] The presence of NDMA in uncooked salted fish was subsequently confirmed by the use of combined gas chromatography and mass spectrometry (GC-MS),[30-32] which is a more specific method for analysis of foodstuffs. When high instead of low resolution mass spectrometry was employed, NDMA in the range of 1 to 35 μg/kg was detected in four of six types of fish samples examined.[33] The detection limit of the method used was 1 μg/kg for each nitrosamine and the quantitative results have a precision of ± 20%.

The presence of nitrosamines in the uncooked salted fish was attributed to their formation by the interaction between nitrite and precursor amines in the fish. The nitrite itself was formed by the reduction by nitrate-reducing *Staphlococcus aureus* of the nitrate present in the crude salt used in the preservation process.[34]

Since the salted fish consumed by southern Chinese is always in the cooked form, it is obviously important that its carcinogenicity should be investigated after the fish has been cooked in the manner it is normally served. Uncooked, steamed, and fried samples were analyzed by gas chromatography with detection by chemiluminescence and some also by combined gas chromatography and high resolution mass spectrometry.[35] NDMA was detected in all the samples that were analyzed, whether cooked or uncooked. It was also detected in the aqueous phase derived from the samples, and in the oil from frying in two of three batches. In one of these the NDMA level was the highest encountered in the study, 2700 ng/ℓ of oil. The highest level of NDMA in the fried samples of fish was 1400 ng/kg and the lowest 200 ng/kg. For the steamed samples the range was 100 to 600 ng/kg and that in the aqueous phase 100 to 400 ng/ℓ. There was often an increased level of NDMA in the cooked samples compared with the uncooked, and NDEA was detected in more batches of the steamed fish than of the uncooked or fried fish. The highest level of NDEA detected in steamed fish samples was only 100 ng/kg and in the aqueous phase 200 ng/ℓ. *N*-nitrosodi-*n*-propylamine (NDPA) was detected in both the steamed and fried samples and *N*-nitrosodi-*n*-butylamine (NDBA) in only the fried samples. Neither was detected in the uncooked samples, whereas *N*-nitrosomorpholine (NMOR) was detected only in the uncooked. These observations confirm that certain nitrosamines are formed from precursors during cooking.[36]

The presence of NDMA and NDEA in the aqueous phase during steaming of salted fish has special significance. It has been the practice among southern Chinese to steam salted fish on top of rice in a cooking utensil with the lid on. This means that some of the aqueous phase containing nitrosamines would find its way into the rice, and that someone might unknowingly take in nitrosamines with the rice without eating the salted fish. It is well-known that exogenous chemicals, including carcinogens, are excreted into the milk during suckling[37] and carcinogens can also pass through the placenta.[38] Consequently, it is important when planning questionnaires for an epidemiological study of NPC to include past histories related to such possibilities. This has been done in an ongoing case-control survey in Hong Kong.

Although it has been established that cooked salted fish is a source of nitrosamines, which are in fact procarcinogens, it has yet to be shown what happens to them after they have entered the body.

A recent evaluation of six short-term tests for predicting carcinogenicity of 120 chemical carcinogens by Purchase et al.[39] concluded that the mutagenicity test developed by Ames et al. using the Salmonella/microsome system had the most extensive application. It is about 90% accurate in detecting a variety of chemical carcinogens as mutagens.[40,41] The Ames test using *Salmonella typhimurium* TA98 and TA100 was employed to detect mutagenic activities in salted fish and in the urine collected from Wistar albino (WA) rats regularly fed steamed cooked salted fish.[42,43] Mutagenic activity toward both tester strains was found in all the salted fish preparations tested and in the urine collected from the experimental rats after salted fish feeding, but the activity decreased markedly in the urine collected after the rats were transferred from a salted fish diet to salted Purina Rat Chow®. It may be presumed that the mutagenic activity in the urine of the experimental rats was derived from their salted fish diet which had caused mutagens to enter the blood circulation and became excreted by the kidneys into the urine. Whether humans would behave similarly on a salted fish diet has yet to be investigated. It would not be unethical to apply the test on southern Chinese adults who had eaten much salted fish in the past.

When Huang et al.[44] fed 10 male and 10 female WA rats steamed salted marine fish as part of their diet for 12 to 24 months, four females developed carcinomas in the nasal or paranasal regions (two developed adenocarcinoma of the nasal cavity, one an undifferentiated carcinoma in a maxillary sinus, and another a highly invasive squamous carcinoma in the right upper bucco-alveolar sulcus). Subsequently, one of two rats similarly fed developed squamous carcinoma of the nasal cavity.[45] None of the control rats developed carcinoma but 3 of 14 given NDEA orally as positive controls developed adenocarcinoma of the nasal cavity. None of the rats and hamsters served as negative controls and also none of the hamsters given the salted fish diet developed nasal or paranasal cancer. Interestingly, although NDMA is the predominant volatile nitrosamine in salted fish, cooked or uncooked, none of 15 rats given NDMA orally developed cancer in the upper respiratory passage.

IV. DISCUSSION AND CONCLUSION

The levels of volatile nitrosamines detected in salted fish, uncooked or cooked, are no higher than those encountered in cured meats consumed in Europe, where the incidence of NPC is low. It is, however, unique in the case of southern Chinese that salted fish is fed to their children from infancy, whereas among Europeans cured meat is usually consumed by older children and adults. The diet of southern Chinese babies during weaning is usually one consisting of fresh or salted fish and practically nothing else added to congee. This lack in variety that might have excluded protective substances, e.g., vitamin C, contained in the diet, the frequency of feeding the same carcinogenic agents, and the greater susceptibility of growing tissue in the young may explain the difference in risk. It may also explain the observations that there was a higher than expected risk of NPC in white males who were born in the Philippines or China of Caucasian stock with no mongoloid admixture,[46] and the development of NPC in three patients of mixed Caucasian (1 British, 1 Norwegian, and 1 Pakistanian) and Chinese marriage who were brought up on a diet predominantly of the Cantonese type.[14]

There is general agreement that NPC has a multifactorial etiology. From epidemiological and experimental data, Ho[14] postulated the involvement of three factors: EBV infection early in life, a genetically determined susceptibility, and environmental factors that vary from population to population. In the case of southern Chinese it would seem that consumption of salted fish at an early age is a major environmental risk factor. If it is, prevention would not be difficult. All that is required is to convince them not to feed their young salted fish. Many of them have already done so, because there are now cheaper and more nutritious foods, such as chicken and milk products, to replace salted fish, which is actually becoming more expensive than chicken, at least in Hong Kong. We would, therefore, have an opportunity to check this hypothesis in 20 to 30 years' time.

REFERENCES

1. **Svoboda, D. J., Kirchner, F. R., and Shanmugaratnam, K.,** The fine structure of nasopharyngeal carcinoma, in *Cancer of the Nasopharynx,* UICC Monogr. Ser. 1, Muir, C. S. and Shanmugaratnam, K., Eds., Munksgaard, Copenhagen, 1967, 163.

2. **Ho, J. H. C.,** Genetic and environmental factors in nasopharyngeal carcinoma, in *Recent Advances in Human Tumour Virology and Immunology,* Proc. 1st Int. Cancer Symp. Princess Takamatsu Cancer Research Fund, Nakahara, W., Nishioka, K., Hirayama, T., and Ito, Y., Eds., University of Tokyo Press, Tokyo, 1971, 275.

3. **Todd, P. J.,** Some practical points in the surgical treatment of cervical tumours, *Chin. Med. J.,* 35, 21, 1921.

4. **Shanmugaratnam, K.,** Studies on the etiology of nasopharyngeal carcinoma, *Int. Rev. Exp. Pathol.,* 10, 361, 1971.

5. **Dobson, W. C.,** Cervical lymphosarcoma, *Chin. Med. J.,* 38, 786, 1924.

6. **Clifford, P. and Beecher, J. L.,** Nasopharyngeal cancer in Kenya. Clinical and environmental aspects, *Br. J. Cancer,* 18, 25, 1964.

7. **Clifford, P.,** Malignant disease of the nasopharynx and paranasal sinuses in Kenya, in *Cancer of the Nasopharynx,* UICC Monograph Series 1, Muir, C. S. and Shanmugaratnam, K., Eds., Munksgaard, Copenhagen, 1967, 82.

8. **Ho, J. H. C.,** Nasopharyngeal carcinoma (NPC), in *Advances in Cancer Research,* Vol. 15, Klein, G., Weinhouse, S., and Haddow, A., Eds., Academic Press, New York, 1972, 57.

9. **Ho, J. H. C.,** Current knowledge of the epidemiology of nasopharyngeal carcinoma — a review, in *Oncogenesis and Herpesviruses,* IARC Sci. Publ. No. 2, Biggs, P. M., de-Thé, G., and Payne, L. N., Eds., International Agency for Research on Cancer, Lyon, France, 1972, 357.

10. **Ho, J. H. C.,** Nasopharyngeal carcinoma in Hong Kong, in *Cancer of the Nasopharynx,* UICC Monograph Series 1, Muir, C. S. and Shanmugaratnam, K., Eds., Munksgaard, Copenhagen, 1967, 29.

11. **Sturton, S. D., Wen, H. L., and Sturton, O. G.,** Etiology of cancer of the nasopharynx, *Cancer,* 19, 1666, 1966.

12. **Ho, J. H. C.,** Epidemiology of nasopharyngeal carcinoma, in *Cancer in Asia, Opportunity for Prevention, Detection and Treatment,* Gann Monograph on Cancer Research, Vol. 18, Hirayama, T., Ed., University of Tokyo Press, Tokyo, 1976, 49.

13. **Ho, J. H. C.,** Epidemiology of nasopharyngeal carcinoma, *J. R. Coll. Surg. Edin.,* 20, 223, 1975.

14. **Ho, J. H. C.,** An epidemiologic and clinical study of nasopharyngeal carcinoma, *Int. J. Rad. Oncol. Biol. Phys.,* 4, 181, 1978.

15. **Topley, M.,** Cultural and social factors relating to Chinese infant feeding and weaning, in *Growing Up in Hong Kong,* Field, C. E. and Barber, F. M., Eds., Hong Kong University Press, Hong Kong, 1973, 56.

16. **Anderson, E. N., Jr., Anderson, M. L., and Ho, J. H. C.,** Environmental backgrounds of young Chinese nasopharyngeal carcinoma patients, in *Nasopharyngeal Carcinoma: Etiology and Control,* IARC Sci. Publ. No. 20, de-Thé, G. and Ito, Y., Eds., International Agency for Research on Cancer, Lyon, France, 1978, 231.

17. **Geser, A., Charney, N., Day, N. E., Ho, J. H. C., and de-Thé, G.,** Environmental factors in the etiology of nasopharyngeal carcinoma: Report on a case-control study in Hong Kong, in *Nasopharyngeal Carcinoma: Etiology and Control,* IARC Sci. Publ. No. 20, de-Thé, G. and Ito, Y., Eds., International Agency for Research on Cancer, Lyon, France, 1978, 213.

18. **Hirayama, T.,** Descriptive and analytical epidemiology of nasopharyngeal cancer, in *Nasopharyngeal Carcinoma: Etiology and Control,* IARC Sci. Publ. No. 20, de-Thé, G. and Ito, Y., Eds., International Agency for Research on Cancer, Lyon, France, 1978, 167.

19. **Lanier, A. P., Bender, T. R., and Talbot, M. L.,** Nasopharyngeal carcinoma in Alaskan Eskimos, Indians, and Aleuts: a review of cases and study of Epstein-Barr virus, HLA, and environmental risk factors, *Cancer,* 46, 2100, 1980.

20. **Yu, M. C., Ho, J. H. C., Ross, R. K., and Henderson, B.,** Nasopharyngeal carcinoma in Chinese salted fish or inhaled smoke? *Prev. Med.,* 10, 15, 1981.

21. **Armstrong, R. W., Armstrong, M. J., Yu, M. C., and Henderson, B.,** Inhalants, salted fish, and nasopharyngeal carcinoma, manuscript in preparation.

22. **Althoff, J., Möhr, U., Page, N., and Reznik, G. J.,** Carcinogenic effect of dibutylnitrosamine in European hamsters *(Cricetus cricetus), J. Natl. Cancer Inst.,* 53, 795, 1974.

23. **Haas, H., Möhr, U., and Kruger, F. W.,** Comparative studies with different doses of N-nitrosomorpholine, N-nitrosopiperidine, N-nitrosomethylurea and dimethylnitrosamine in Syrian golden hamsters, *J. Natl. Cancer Inst.,* 51, 1295, 1973.

24. **Pour, P., Kruger, F. W., Cardesa, A., Althoff, J., and Möhr, U.,** Carcinogenic effect of d-n-propyl-nitrosamine in Syrian golden hamsters, *J. Natl. Cancer Inst.,* 51, 1019, 1973.

25. **Cardesa, A., Pour, P., Haas, H., Althoff, J., and Möhr, U.,** Histogenesis of tumors from the nasal cavities induced by DEN, *Cancer,* 37, 346, 1976.
26. **Pelfrene, A. and Garcia, H.,** Chemically induced esthesioneuroblastomas in rats, *Z. Krebsforsch.,* 86, 113, 1976.
27. **Lijinsky, W.,** How nitrosamines cause cancer, *New Scientist,* 73, 216, 1977.
28. **Fong, Y. Y. and Walsh, E. O. F.,** Carcinogenic nitrosamines in Cantonese salt-dried fish, *Lancet,* 2, 1032, 1971.
29. **Sen, N. P., Smith, D. C., Schwinghamer, L., and Marleau, J. J.,** Diethylnitrosamine and other N-nitrosamines in food, *J. Assoc. Off. Anal. Chem.,* 52, 47, 1969.
30. **Fong, Y. Y. and Chan, W. C.,** Dimethylnitrosamine in Chinese marine salt fish, *Food Cosmet. Toxicol.,* 11, 841, 1973.
31. *Report of the Government Chemist 1973,* Her Majesty's Stationery Office, London, England, 1974, 45.
32. **Fong, Y. Y. and Chan, W. C.,** Methods for limiting the content of di-methylnitrosamine in Chinese marine salt fish, *Food Cosmet. Toxicol.,* 14, 95, 1976.
33. **Huang, D. P., Ho, J. H. C., Gough, T. A., and Webb, K. S.,** Volatile nitrosamines in some traditional southern Chinese food products, *J. Food Safety,* 1, 1, 1977.
34. **Fong, Y. Y. and Chan, W. C.,** Bacterial production of dimethylnitrosamine in salted fish, *Nature (London),* 243, 421, 1973.
35. **Huang, D. P., Ho, J. H. C., Webb, K. S., Wood, B. J., and Gough, T. A.,** Volatile nitrosamines in salt preserved fish, before and after cooking, *Food Cosmet. Toxicol.,* 19, 167, 1981.
36. **Gough, T. A., Webb, K. S., and Coleman, R. F.,** Estimate of the volatile nitrosamine content of the U.K. food, *Nature (London),* 272, 161, 1978.
37. **Ing, R., Ho, J. H. C., and Petrakis, N. L.,** Unilateral breast-feeding and breast cancer, *Lancet,* 2, 124, 1977.
38. Editorial, Transplacental carcinogenesis, *Lancet,* 1, 1425, 1973.
39. **Purchase, I. F. H., Longstapf, E., Ashby, J., Styles, J. A., Anderson, D., Lefevre, P. A., and Westwood, F. R.,** An evaluation of six short-tests for detecting organic chemical carcinogens, *Br. J. Cancer,* 37, 873, 1978.
40. **Ames, B. N., McCann, J., and Yamasaki, E.,** Methods for detecting carcinogens and mutagens with the *Salmonella*/mammalian microsome mutagenicity test, *Mutat. Res.,* 31, 347, 1975.
41. **McCann, J., Choi, E., Yamasaki, E., and Ames, B. N.,** Detection of carcinogens as mutagens in the *Salmonella*/microsome test: assay of 300 chemicals, *Proc. Natl. Acad. Sci. U.S.A.,* 72, 5135, 1975.
42. **Ho, J. H. C., Huang, D. P., and Fong, Y. Y.,** Salted fish and nasopharyngeal carcinoma in southern Chinese, *Lancet,* 2, 626, 1978.
43. **Fong, L. Y. Y., Huang, D. P., and Ho, J. H. C.,** Preserved foods as possible cancer hazards: WA rats fed salted fish have mutagenic urine, *Int. J. Cancer,* 23, 542, 1979.
44. **Huang, D. P., Saw, D., Teoh, T. B., and Ho, J. H. C.,** Carcinoma of nasal and paranasal regions in rats fed Cantonese salted fish, in *Nasopharyngeal Carcinoma; : Etiology and Control,* IARC Sci. Publ. No. 20, de-Thé, G. and Ito, Y., Eds., International Agency for Research on Cancer, Lyon, France, 1978, 315.
45. **Huang, D. P., Ho, H. C., and Chan, W. C.,** unpublished data, 1978.
46. **Buell, P.,** Race and place in the etiology of nasopharyngeal cancer: a study based on Californian death certificates, *Int. J. Cancer,* 11, 268, 1973.

Chapter 4

MUTAGENIC COMPONENTS OF DIETS IN HIGH- AND LOW-RISK AREAS FOR STOMACH CANCER

Sigetosi Kamiyama and Osamu Michioka

TABLE OF CONTENTS

I. INTRODUCTION

Deaths from malignant neoplasms in Japan[1] have increased by about 3500 annually for the last 10 years, and reached 150,000 in 1978. This was 21.6% of total deaths and ranked as the second main cause after cerebrovascular diseases. By 1981, cerebrovascular diseases had taken second place. Estimating by 5-year age classes, cancer deaths ranked first in all classes from 30 to 74. This means that a person of working age in Japan is now facing significant cancer risks.

With respect to site, stomach cancer is the most prevalent in Japan for both males and females. In 1978, stomach cancer was about 35 and 30% for males and females, respectively, of total cancer deaths. These percentages are very different from country to country, and in U.S. whites were only 4.1% for males and 2.6% for females for the period 1969 to 1971.[2] In addition, the fact that stomach cancer deaths among Japanese immigrants to Hawaii and California[3] decrease to the level of the U.S. population suggests that the environment has a very large influence on stomach cancer mortality.

The phenomenon of regional aggregation in stomach cancer mortality[4] is also observed. High-risk areas are seen in the prefectures of Akita, Yamagata, Niigata, Toyama, and Ishikawa, all located on the Japan Sea side of northern Honshu, the Japanese mainland. The other high-risk areas are in the prefectures of Nara and Wakayama in the southern Kinki area of the central part of the mainland. On the other hand, low-risk areas are seen on the Pacific Ocean side of northern Honshu, including Iwate and Aomori prefectures, and also in the southern part of Kyushu island, including Kagoshima, Kumamoto, and Miyazaki prefectures (Figure 1).

It is striking that high and low stomach cancer mortalities are found in the Akita and Iwate prefectures which are separated only by the central mountain range. Every year the stomach cancer mortality in the Akita prefecture, which is located on the Japan Sea side, ranks in the highest group, and that in Iwate, which is located on the Pacific Ocean side, ranks in the lowest group. We have carried out studies to elucidate the cause of the different mortalities between the two prefectures.

For this purpose, two farm villages, one from each prefecture, were selected for the survey. The geographical and geological features, the genetic traits, and dietary habits of the inhabitants, and the daily drinking water were compared.[5] A cooked meal from each surveyed person was collected and homogenized each day, then subjected to the mutagenicity tests of the rec-assay and the Ames test. The results[6] revealed a large difference in the mutagenicity of the diets between the two districts, Akita being high and Iwate low, corresponding to the difference in the stomach cancer mortalities.

II. SUBJECTS AND METHODS

A. Summary of the Survey Locations

As described above, Chokai village (Akita village) and Ohasama Town (Iwate village) were selected as the survey locations for the high- and low-risk areas. The population, according to the 1975 national census, of the Akita village was 9085 (4539 males and 4546 females) in 2074 households, and that of the Iwate village was 8555 (4165 males and 4390 females) in 2072 households. The geographies and socioeconomic levels were very similar in the two places. The age-adjusted mortalities from stomach cancer per 100,000 population in each 5-year period for 1968 to 1972 were 60.0 for males and 32.1 for females in Akita village, and 25.5 for males and 14.2 for females in Iwate village, standardized to the general Japanese population of 1960. The cerebrovascular mortalities of the two locations were high compared to the national average.

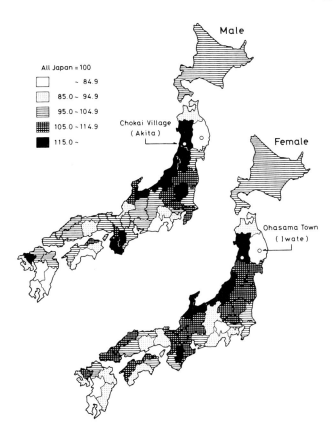

FIGURE 1.   Ratios of age-adjusted death rates for stomach cancer in Japan in 1975 (standard population:total population of Japan in 1960).

B. Dietary Survey

A dietary survey was carried out, using a self-recorded system, of cooked foods taken in a day by a randomly selected 20 males and 11 females in Akita and by 25 males and 11 females in Iwate. The subjects recorded the menus of each meal of the day; the names of foods used; the number of dishes, bowls, or cups, including snacks or between-meals; and beverages. From these descriptions, intakes of energy, protein, iron, calcium, and vitamins A and C were calculated by the method of Fukui and Nakata.[7] A comparison between the average values of these nutritional intakes was made for the two villages. The amounts of cooked foods were also calculated and compared by an χ^2-test between the two locations.

A similar dietary survey was carried out for housewives in both villages for two days in every month for 12 months. Seasonal variation in dietary intake was followed using 4509 and 2586 meals, respectively, in the Akita and the Iwate villages. The results have been described by Shimada[8] elsewhere.

C. Mutagenicity Tests of Different Diets

In Japan, the following two kinds of bacterial mutagenicity tests are widely used. One is the rec-assay, which detects the repair efficiency of damaged DNA in *subtilis* bacteria, and the other is the Ames test which estimates the revertant induction in Salmonella by chemical mutagens. Both tests were used in our study.

Twenty-six (26) and 36 households, respectively, were randomly selected in the Akita and Iwate villages, and male or female householders were used. Cooked foods that corresponded to each meal ingested by the subject were collected for one day. The foods were kept in a refrigerator until collected. The collected foods were transported chilled to our laboratory and stored frozen.

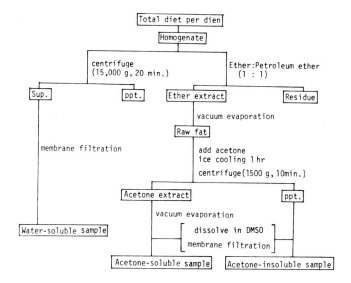

FIGURE 2.   Procedure for preparation of samples for mutagenicity tests.

The edible portions of the thawed dietary specimens for each person per day were weighed and homogenized in a large Waring blender. The pastes were stored frozen for chemical and mutagenic analyses. As seen in Figure 2, each sample was extracted with a mixture of petroleum and ethyl ethers (1:1 by volume), and the extract concentrated to dryness in an evaporator (raw fat fraction). This fraction was tested by the rec-assay using *Bacillus subtilis* H15 and M45 by Kada's method.[9]

The raw fat fraction was again extracted with cold acetone and the acetone-soluble fraction concentrated to dryness in a vacuum freeze-dryer and then subjected to the Ames test[10] using *Salmonella typhimurium* TA98 and TA100 after preincubation[11] with S9 mix. To induce the metabolic enzyme PCB (KC-500) was given i.p. to Sprague-Dawley rats.

As a positive control for the mutagenicity tests, 2-acetylaminofluorene (AAF) or benzo[a]pyrene (BaP) was used after being dissolved in dimethyl sulfoxide (DMSO) and preincubated with S9 mix. The DMSO which was used to dissolve the specimens and the positive controls served as the negative control with S9 mix. The revertant colonies were counted using an automatic colony counter (Biotran Model II).

To estimate mutagenicity in the Ames test using TA100 and TA98, the number of revertant colonies was divided by that of the negative control. The relative mutation ratios were then divided into three grades, greater than 3, 3 to 1.5, and less than 1.5. These were called positive, probable, and negative mutagenicities.

The frequencies of the positive, the probable, and the negative mutagenicities were calculated for the specimens tested in the two villages. The frequency of appearance of cooked foods was then compared among the positive, the probable, and the negative diet groups. The foods which appeared significantly more often ($p < 0.05$) in the positive mutagenic diet were called the mutagen-positive food group. Similarly, the foods which appeared significantly more often ($p < 0.05$) in the negative mutagenic diet were called the mutagen-negative food group.

D. Mutagenicity and Mutagen-Depressing Tests of Foods

To conduct the mutagenicity and the mutagen-depressing tests, five households each were selected from those eating the mutagen-positive diet, the mutagen-probable diet, and the mutagen-negative diet. They were asked to prepare the same kinds of meals according to the menus of the previous survey. At the same time, the raw materials used in the cooking were also collected. The foods, cooked and raw, were subjected to the Ames test using *Salmonella typhimurium* TA100 as described above.

Table 1
MUTAGEN-DEPRESSIVE EFFECT OF
VEGETABLES

	DMSO	Onion (500 mg)	Cabbage (500 mg)
Control (DMSO)	100	116	124
BaP (5 μg)	275	149	118
AAF (10 μg)	368	96	78
3-MC (5 μg)	338	115	146

In each case, 5 g of food paste was used as the starting material, and the acetone-soluble fraction was dissolved in DMSO and made up to 2.5 mℓ. This extract was sterilized by filtering through a Millipore filter. The solution was diluted to 1, 5, and 25 times using sterilized DMSO, and each concentration was preincubated with S9 mix before testing.

To show the mutagen-depressing effects of food materials, acetone-soluble fractions were extracted from 10 g of onion or cabbage by the same procedures. The fractions were dissolved in DMSO and made up to 1 mℓ. Then 50 μℓ of the solution, which corresponds to 500 mg of the starting materials, was mixed with the same volume of a DMSO solution of BaP (100 μg/mℓ), AAF (200 μg/mℓ) or 3-MC (20-methylcholanthrene, 100 μg/mℓ), and also with DMSO as the negative control; 100 μℓ of solution corresponded to 5 μg, 10 μg, and 5 μg of BaP, AAF, and 3-MC, respectively. Depressant effects on the development of the revertant colonies were detected, as shown in Table 1. Since the greatest effect of both materials was seen on AAF, this chemical was used as the indicator of the mutagen-depressing effect of foods.

E. Intake of Mutagen-Related Foods

The results of the mutagenicity and the mutagen-depressing tests on each food, cooked and raw, revealed that there was a pattern. Mutagenic effects are greatest in broiled meat, grilled fish, and salted fish guts, but weak in cooked beans, fried bean curd, sauteed vegetables, salted wild plants, and sauteed onions. Mutagen-depressing effects were strong in fresh vegetables, fresh Western vegetables, and potatoes, but weak or hardly detectable in cooked carrots, milk, soybean curd, konjac (devil's tongue), and confections. From these results, an attempt was made to evaluate the combined mutagenic and mutagen-depressing effects of particular diets. For food items which show strong mutagenicity or which have a strong mutagen-depressing effect, points were given equal in number to the times that the food item appeared in all the meals in a day. For foods which have weak effects, only one point was given regardless of the number of times an item appeared during a day. Separate overall scores, one for mutagen-positive and one for mutagen-negative food items in each diet belonging to the mutagen-positive, the mutagen-probable, and the mutagen-negative diet groups, were calculated and then plotted on a rectangular diagonal. The range of their distributions was expressed as a probability ellipse of 95% critical regions for each diet group.

III. RESULTS AND DISCUSSION

A. Regional Differences in Food Intake

The frequencies of appearance of most food items in the diets were higher in the Iwate village. This was seen especially for vegetables. Among animal foods, both groups of inhabitants took their highest intake in eggs with no significant difference between them. Salted fish was eaten very often in Akita. In addition, miso (fermented salty bean paste) was taken more frequently in Akita. However, there were no significant differences in the

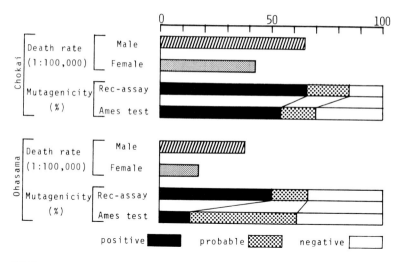

FIGURE 3.   Age-adjusted stomach cancer mortalities and mutagenicity of diets in the Akita (Chokai) and the Iwate (Ohasama) villages.

frequencies of appearance of tofu (soybean curd) and natto (fermented soybean). Male inhabitants of Akita ate cooked rice, miso, sake (Japanese rice brew), pickled eggplants, and sweet potatoes significantly more often than Iwate inhabitants in November. Males and females in the Iwate village seemed to eat carrots, Welsh onions, seaweeds, and cooked rice with barley more often.

B. Mutagenicity of Diets

The results in the rec-assay produced by the raw fat fractions extracted from the homogenized pastes of daily diets of different persons showed large differences in the degree of positive mutagenicity. With or without S9 mix, the positive scores were significantly higher for diets from the Akita village.

The results of Ames tests using Salmonella TA100 and TA98 on acetone-soluble fractions also revealed that there were marked differences between the two districts in the relative mutagenicities similar to those revealed by the rec-assay.

The mutation ratios were divided into three grades: positive, probable, and negative, as described already in the methods section. The results are shown in Figure 3. The frequency of positive test scores was significantly higher in Akita than in Iwate.

The results of the mutagenicity tests clearly show that the diets taken by the inhabitants of the Akita village contain more mutagenic components than those taken by the inhabitants of the Iwate village.

C. Frequency of Appearance of Foods in Different Mutagenicity Groups

The results from the Akita and Iwate districts of mutagenicity tests using Salmonella TA100 were combined and analyzed according to food intake. The diets were divided according to mutagenicity scores into three groups: the positive, the probable, and the negative mutagenic groups. The number of daily diets in each group was 19, 21, and 22, respectively. Each cooked food item was tallied and grouped according to its nature and cooking method, and the frequency of its appearance was described as a percentage of the total number of diets.

In general, the major differences between the mutagenic diet groups could be accounted for by the proteinaceous foods and vegetables. A comparison between the frequencies of appearance of particular foods was made pairwise between the mutagen-positive, the mutagen-probable, and the mutagen-negative diet groups to identify the mutagenic components in the diets.

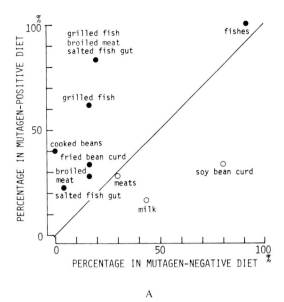

FIGURE 4. Frequencies of food appearance in the mutagen-positive and the mutagen-negative diet groups. (A) Protein foods; (B) vegetable foods.

In Figure 4A and B are shown two examples of the frequency of appearance of protein-aceous and vegetable foods within the mutagen-positive and the mutagen-negative groups. Among the proteinaceous foods, there were no differences between the two diet groups in the overall frequencies of appearance of fish and meat. However, broiled meats, grilled fish, salted fish guts, and cooked beans seemed to appear more often in the mutagen-negative diet group. When the frequencies of appearance of broiled meats, grilled fish, and salted fish guts were combined, the frequency of appearance of these foods exceeds 80% in the mutagen-positive diets, whereas the frequency of these foods is only 15% in the mutagen-negative diets. Comparison between the mutagen-positive and the mutagen-probable diet groups showed essentially similar frequencies of appearance, except that soybean curd is significantly more frequent in the latter group. However, comparison between the mutagen-probable and the mutagen-negative diet groups showed a very similar pattern to that of the mutagen-positive and mutagen-negative diet groups, especially in that the total frequency of broiled meats, grilled fish, and salted fish guts was significantly larger in the mutagen-probable diet group.

On the other hand, a similar study of vegetable foods required that account be taken of the cooking methods used. The mutagenicity of vegetables varies very much according to how they are cooked. We divided the cooked vegetable foods into four kinds: (A) fresh, (B) salted or pickled, (C) sauteed, and (D) boiled. As an example, Figure 4B shows the comparison between the mutagen-positive and mutagen-negative diet groups. In general, vegetable foods appeared more frequently in the mutagen-negative diet group. In the mutagen-positive diet group, salted vegetables, sauteed onions, and salted wild plants such as bracken fern appeared significantly more often, whereas fresh vegetables and fresh Western vegetables appeared more frequently in the mutagen-negative diet group. Confections were also more frequent in the latter group, but almost all of them seem to be made from cereals such as rice cake. The frequent appearance of specific foods in different groups reveals a recognizable pattern. Comparison between the mutagen-positive and mutagen-probable diet groups showed a fairly similar pattern to that of the above-mentioned relationship between the mutagen-positive and mutagen-negative diet groups, although sauteed onions and salted wild plants appeared more often in the mutagen-positive diets, and fresh vegetables, potatoes, and cooked carrots were significantly more frequent in the mutagen-probable diet group. The frequencies of appearance in the mutagen-probable and mutagen-negative diet groups were essentially the same.

Based on these observations, the class of foods which showed up significantly more often in the mutagen-positive diets than in the other two diet groups was called the mutagen-positive food group. Correspondingly, the food group which showed up significantly more often in the mutagen-negative diets was called the mutagen-negative food group. The foods found in the mutagen-positive group were broiled meats, grilled fish, salted fish guts, cooked beans, fried bean curd, sauteed vegetables, salted wild plants, and sauteed onions, as shown in Figure 5. The foods in the mutagen-negative group were fresh vegetables, fresh Western vegetables, cooked carrots, milk, soybean curd, konjac (mannan or devil's tongue), and confections.

D. Comparison of Mutagenicity of Foods

1. Mutagenicity and Mutagen-Depressing Effects in the Mutagen-Positive Food Group

Acetone-soluble fractions of the cooked foods belonging to the mutagen-positive group and their raw materials were subjected to the Ames test using Salmonella TA100. These food samples were prepared at each of the five households that offered mutagen-positive, mutagen-probable, and mutagen-negative diets in the two survey locations. At the same time, possible mutagen-depressing effects of the same acetone-soluble fractions of cooked foods and their raw materials were tested for by the Ames TA100 method after adding 10 μg AAF as the standard mutagen. The results of both the mutagenicity and the mutagen-depressing tests were expressed as the ratio of the mean revertant colonies to the negative control (DMSO) expressed as 100, as shown in Table 2.

Cooked foods, such as broiled meats, grilled fish, and salted fish guts, showed strong mutagenicity. However, broiled mutton, cabbage, and onions showed no mutagenicity and even had a large mutagen-depressing effect on AAF. Sauteed vegetables showed only slight mutagenicity and, except for sauteed sweet peppers, also some mutagen-depressing effect.

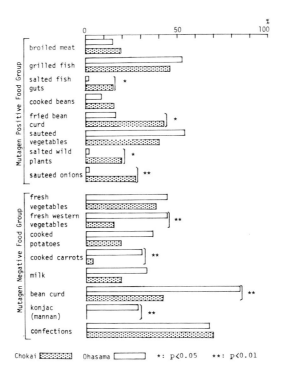

FIGURE 5. Mutagen-positive and mutagen-negative food groups, and frequencies of intake in all meals per day in the Akita and Iwate villages.

On the other hand, raw food materials showed almost no mutagenicity. Semi-processed food materials, such as salted trout and smoked bonito, showed both mutagenicity and an enhancing effect on the mutagenicity of AAF. Smoked bonito used as a cooking material is mutagenic and also increases the mutagenicity of AAF when it is dressed with liquid starch. However, mutagenicity disappeared and the mutagen-depressing effect appeared when it was hashed with cucumber and vinegar. This shows that major differences are produced by different cooking methods, even when the same food material is used as a main component. Food materials of animal origin have almost no enhancing effect on the mutagenicity of AAF, with the exception described above. Except for sweet pepper, vegetables showed very strong depressive effects.

2. Mutagenicity and Mutagen-Depressing Effects in the Mutagen-Negative Food Group

Table 3 shows the results of the mutagenicity and mutagen-depressing tests carried out on each food item belonging to the mutagen-negative group. Slightly positive mutagenicity was observed in sweet pepper, parsley, and baked rice cake with sesame, and in addition a bacteriocidal effect was seen in konjac (devil's tongue). Other foods produced almost the same levels of revertants as the DMSO control. On the other hand, mutagen-depressing effects were seen in almost all the vegetable foods except garlic, sweet pepper, and parsley. Milk, soybean curd, and rice cake with sesame did not clearly show any depressive effects on the mutagenicity of AAF. The mutagen-depressive effect of potatoes weakened slightly when they were fried in oil.

3. Changes in Mutagenicity and Mutagen-Depressing Effects Induced by Cooking

The above-mentioned tests of the mutagenicity of broiled mutton with onions and smoked bonito with hashed cucumber indicate the appearance of mutagen-depressing effects during

Table 2
MUTAGENICITY OF COOKED FOOD AND RAW MATERIAL

Cooked food	Added food/plate (mg)	DMSO	AAF 10 μg	Raw material	Added food/plate (mg)	DMSO	AAF 10 μg
Control (DMSO)		100	368			100	368
Broiled meat							
Broiled pork	50	279	468	Pork	50	121	294
Broiled mutton	50	74	292	Mutton	50	102	388
Grilled fish							
Grilled horse mackerel	10	284	713	Horse mackerel	50	117	356
Grilled sardine	10	398	830	Sardine	50	96	419
Grilled salt trout	2	327	822	Salt trout	10	213	795
Smoked bonito with hashed cucumber seasoned with vinegar	50	79	146	Smoked bonito	10	293	534
Smoked bonito dressed with liquid starch	50	282	431				
Cooked bean							
Cooked black soybean	50	148	366	Black soybean	50	143	317
Salted fish guts							
Salted bonito guts	10	347	838				
Salted cuttlefish guts	2	392	780				
Salted wild plants							
Salted bracken	50	102	372				
Sauteed vegetables							
Sweet pepper	50	149	388	Sweet pepper	50	148	373
Carrot	50	133	214	Carrot	50	131	95
Cabbage	50	124	192	Cabbage	50	126	102
Onion	50	108	184	Onion	50	114	89
Fried bean curd	50	138	396	Soybean curd	50	106	272

the course of cooking. In addition, mutagen-depressing effects were weakened after sauteeing or frying. These observations led us to conduct experiments to follow changes in mutagenicity and the mutagen-depressing effect of cabbage induced by cooking.

Samples of fresh and sauteed cabbage were homogenized separately and extracted by the usual procedure to yield two acetone-soluble fractions. These two samples were successively diluted with DMSO, and fractions corresponding to 500, 250, 125, 62.5, or 31.25 mg of the original food material were added to the plates. The results are shown in Table 4. Slight mutagenicity was seen at the 500 mg of fresh cabbage, but not at other dilutions. The mutagen-depressing effect was very strong at every dilution, with a gradual decrease only noticeable at 2^3 and 2^4 times dilutions, corresponding to 62.5 mg and 31.25 mg of the original material.

On the other hand, sauteed cabbage showed very low mutagenicity at almost all dilutions, except for the highest (2^4 times). The mutagen-depressing effects were weaker than those from fresh material at every dilution. The highest dilution (2^4 times) produced more than twice the number of revertant colonies than the raw material. This shows that the mutagen-depressing effect is weakened by sauteeing.

E. Combined Intake of Mutagen-Related Foods

The results from the tests described above on the mutagenic and mutagen-depressing effects in the mutagen-positive and mutagen-negative food groups revealed the need to evaluate their combined effects using weighted criteria. Table 5 shows weighted criteria for both the mutagenic and mutagen-depressing effects of the various food items.

Table 3
DEPRESSIVE EFFECTS OF MUTAGEN-
NEGATIVE FOODS ON AAF

	Added food/ plate (mg)	DMSO	AAF 10 μg
Control (DMSO)		100	368
Cucumber	50	96	123
Onion	50	114	89
Cabbage	50	126	102
Chinese radish	50	104	118
Radish	50	122	115
Garlic	10	84	289
Sweet pepper	50	148	373
Lettuce	50	92	98
Celery	50	106	103
Parsley	50	168	370
Konjak (mannan)	10	84	207
Potatoes	50	109	104
Fried potatoes	50	110	136
Carrot	50	131	95
Milk	50	133	341
Soybean curd	50	106	272
Baked rice cake with sesame	50	149	306

Table 4
CHANGE IN MUTAGEN-DEPRESSIVE EFFECT OF
CABBAGE BY SAUTEEING

	Raw cabbage		Sauteed cabbage	
Added food/plate (mg)	DMSO	AAF 10 μg	DMSO	AAF 10 μg
Control (DMSO)	100	368	100	368
500	124	78	107	98
250	80	86	101	108
125	96	72	111	148
62.5	92	102	98	162
31.25	81	112	124	248

Table 5
EVALUATION OF COMBINED MUTAGENIC AND MUTAGEN-
DEPRESSIVE EFFECTS OF FOODS: CRITERIA USED

Mutagen-positive food group	Standard of evaluation	Mutagen-negative food group
Broiled meats	Points are given according	Fresh vegetable
Grilled fish	to the frequency of ap-	Fresh western vegetables
Salted fish guts	pearance in meals of one day	Potatoes
Cooked beans	One point is given when	Cooked carrots
Fried soybean curd	the food appeared in meals of a day, regardless of the frequency	Milk
Sauteed vegetables		Soybean curd
Salted wild plants		Konjac (devil's tongue)
Sauteed onions		Confections

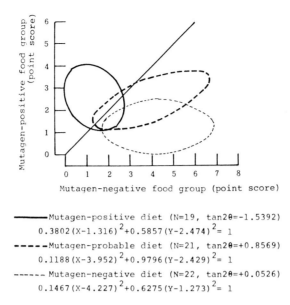

—————Mutagen-positive diet (N=19, tan2θ=-1.5392)
$0.3802(X-1.316)^2+0.5857(Y-2.474)^2= 1$

- - - - -Mutagen-probable diet (N=21, tan2θ=+0.8569)
$0.1188(X-3.952)^2+0.9796(Y-2.429)^2= 1$

- - - - - - Mutagen-negative diet (N=22, tan2θ=+0.0526)
$0.1467(X-4.227)^2+0.6275(Y-1.273)^2= 1$

FIGURE 6.   Patterns of food intake according to mutagenic characteristics, shown by probability ellipses of 95% critical regions.

Using these weighted values, two scores were calculated for each diet, one for the mutagen-positive items and one for the mutagen-negative items. The distributions of these twin scores were plotted for 19, 21, and 22 samples, respectively, in the mutagen-positive, mutagen-probable, and mutagen-negative diet groups. The range of the distributions was expressed as a probability ellipse of 95% critical values (Figure 6). The distribution of the twin scores for all mutagen-positive diets correlates with the mutagen-positive food group and conversely the scores for the mutagen-negative diets with the mutagen-negative food group. The scores for the mutagen-probable diets are distributed between the other two groups.

In daily life, meals are the most important occasion to take up foreign substances into the human body. Especially since they may be possible factors in causing GI cancers, foods have been the subject of great concern, both in experimental and epidemiological studies. From these studies, certain *N*-nitroso compounds,[12] polycyclic aromatic hydrocarbons,[13] and mycotoxins[14] have been identified as carcinogenic substances in animal experiments. However, these substances are not, by themselves, sufficient to explain the main causation of human cancer and especially not of stomach cancer.

Recent developments in the study of mutagenesis have provided practical tests for screening of mutagenic and carcinogenic substances. Sugimura and Nagao[15] have summarized their studies on the mutagenic factors in foods by the extensive application of the Ames test using *Salmonella typhimurium* TA100 and TA98. They especially investigated the pyrolysis products of proteinaceous foods and amino acids, and discovered such strongly mutagenic and also carcinogenic substances as Trp-P-1, Trp-P-2, Glu-P-1, and IQ. However, these mutagenic substances from the pyrolysates of foods produced cancer only in the liver and not in the stomach.

In our study, broiled or grilled foods also showed strong mutagenicity. However, this mutagenicity is weakened when these foods are taken with such mutagenicity-depressing items as vegetables. Many case-control studies[16] and cohort studies[17] have shown the negative association between stomach cancer and the intake of fresh vegetables. Our mutagenicity study of foods may have closed the gap between the observations of stomach cancer occurrence and the diets consumed.

IV. CONCLUSIONS

This study began with an epidemiological point of view and has led to the classification of foods into two groups: the mutagen-positive and the mutagen-negative group. The difference in pattern of intake between these two groups of foods conveniently explains the different risks of stomach cancer observed in Japan, not only between the Akita and the Iwate villages described in this paper, but also between the other high- and low-risk areas[18] of Nara and Kagoshima.

The results obtained suggest the possibility of the prevention of stomach cancer through controlled dietary habits.

ACKNOWLEDGMENTS

The authors wish to express their thanks for the support of the Cancer Research Fund and the Scientific Research Fund from the Ministry of Education, Cancer Research Support from the Ministry of Health and Welfare, and the Japan-Hawaii Cancer Study, NCI Contract No. NO1 CP61060.

REFERENCES

1. Health and Welfare Statistics Association, *Trends of Nation's Health (Japanese)*, Tokyo, 1981.
2. **Segi, M. and Kurihara, M.,** *Cancer Mortality for Selected Sites in 24 Countries, No. 6 (1966—1967),* Japan Cancer Society, Tokyo, 1979.
3. **Haenszel, W. and Kurihara, M.,** Studies of Japanese migrants. I. Mortality from cancer and other diseases among Japanese in the United States, *J. Natl. Cancer Inst.,* 40, 43, 1968.
4. *Atlas of Cancer Mortality for Japan by Cities and Counties, 1969—1971,* Daiwa Health Foundation, Tokyo, 1977.
5. **Kamiyama, S.,** Risk factors of stomach cancer from metabolic aspects, in *Cancers, Japan and the World,* Nagayo, T. and Tominaga, S., Eds., Shinohara Shuppan Company, Tokyo, 1980, 257.
6. **Kamiyama, S.,** Studies on regional difference of gastric cancer mortality and dietary mutagenicity, *Akita J. Med.,* 7, 227, 1981.
7. **Fukui, T. and Nakata, H.,** A simplified method of the nutritional survey in agricultural districts, *Shikoku Acta Med.,* 27, 385, 1971.
8. **Shimada, A.,** A study on dietary habits of populations in Akita and Iwate prefectures with different gastric cancer risks, *Akita J. Med.,* 7, 153, 1980.
9. **Kada, T., Tsutikawa, K., and Sadaie, Y.,** *In vitro* and host-mediated "rec-assay" procedures for screening chemical mutagens, and phloxine, a mutagenic red dye detected, *Mutat. Res.,* 16, 165, 1972.
10. **Ames, B. N., McCann, J., and Yamasaki, E.,** Methods for detecting carcinogens and mutagens with the *Salmonella*/mammalian-microsome mutagenicity test, *Mutat. Res.,* 31, 347, 1975.
11. **Sugimura, T., Yahagi, T., Nagao, M., Takeuchi, M., Kawachi, T., Hara, K., Yamasaki, E., Matsushima, T., Hashimoto, Y., and Okada, M.,** Validity of mutagenicity tests using microbes as a rapid screening method for environmental carcinogens, in *Screening Tests in Chemical Carcinogenesis,* Tomatis, L., Montesano, R., and Bartsch, H., Eds., IARC Sci. Publ. No. 12, International Agency for Research on Cancer, Lyon, France, 1976, 81.
12. **Magee, P. N. and Barnes, J. M.,** Carcinogenic nitroso-compounds, in *Advances in Cancer Research,* Vol. 10, Haddow, A. and Weinhouse, S., Eds., Academic Press, New York, 1973, 163.
13. IARC Monographs on the Evaluation of Carcinogenic Risk of Chemicals to Man, Vol. 3, *Certain Polycyclic Aromatic Hydrocarbons and Heterocyclic Compounds,* International Agency for Research on Cancer, Lyon, France, 1973.
14. **Purchase, I. F. H.,** *Symposium on Mycotoxins in Human Health,* Macmillan, London, 1971.
15. **Sugimura, T. and Nagao, N.,** Mutagenic factors in cooked foods, *CRC Crit. Rev. Toxicol.,* 189, 1979.

16. **Haenszel, W., Kurihara, M., Segi, M., and Lee, R. K. C.,** Stomach cancer among Japanese in Hawaii, *J. Natl. Cancer Inst.,* 49, 969, 1972.

17. **Hirayama, T.,** A large-scale cohort study on the relationship between diet and selected cancers of digestive organs, in *Gastrointestinal Cancer: Endogenous Factors,* Banbury Report 7, Bruce, W. R., Correa, P., Lipkin, M., Tannenbaum, S. R., and Wilkins, T. D., Eds., Cold Spring Harbor Laboratory, Cold Spring Harbor, N.Y., 1981, 409.

18. **Kamiyama, S., Michioka, O., and Kudo, K.,** Patterns of food intake in four areas of different risks of stomach cancer in viewpoint of mutagenicity, *Proc. Jpn. Cancer Assoc.,* 412, 1981.

Chapter 5

THE ROLE OF SALIVA-BORNE MUTAGENS AND CARCINOGENS IN THE ETIOLOGY OF ORAL AND ESOPHAGEAL CARCINOMAS OF BETEL NUT AND TOBACCO CHEWERS

Hans F. Stich, Bruce A. Bohm, Kamalesh Chatterjee, and J. L. Sailo

TABLE OF CONTENTS

I. PROBLEM

For centuries numerous plant products have been chewed by many different population groups. Among them, the betel nut *(Areca catechu)*, tobacco *(Nicotiana tabacum)*, betel leaf *(Piper betle)*, and miang leaf (wild tea) have become the best known examples because of their suspected role in the etiology of oral, pharyngeal, and esophageal cancers. Among the Indian population, about 70% of cancers of the oral cavity, 75% of cancers of the hypopharynx and larynx, and 50% of esophageal cancers appear to be due to "pan" chewing and/or tobacco smoking.[1] A change in this habit could lead to a drastic reduction of these cancers. Unfortunately, the chewing of betel nut and lime continues unabated among the hill tribes of the northeastern region of India and among the Papuans of Papua New Guinea. The use of "pan", consisting of tobacco, betel nut, betel leaf, seeds, perfumes, and lime, has been only slightly reduced among members of the younger population segment in southern India, Malaysia, and Sri Lanka. However, the chewing of carcinogen-containing plant products is not restricted to Asiatic countries. Snuff dipping is still a common practice among rural women in southeastern regions of the U.S.[2] It seems to be responsible for an elevated risk for cancer of the gum and buccal mucosa.[3] Of particular concern, however, is the rapidly increasing popularity of tobacco chewing among teenagers of European and American countries, leading to the prediction of a new age for snuff.[4]

Considering the number of current investigations and published papers on the etiology of oral and pharyngeal carcinomas, one arrives at the conclusion that this particular cancer problem does not receive the attention it appears to deserve. The percentage contribution of oral cancer to total cancer prevalence is, however, not negligible: it amounts to 75.9% in Neyyur, 67.9% in Mainpuri, 66.1% in Jaffua,[5] about 50% in Bombay,[6] and 23% for males in Papua New Guinea.[7] The seriousness of the various chewing habits can also be deduced from relative risk data of cancers at specific sites. Among "pan"-chewing Indians, the risk of developing oral cancers is between 12 and 18 times higher than among nonchewers, and more than 60 times higher in individuals who retain the quid in the mouth throughout the sleeping period.[8,9] Among American snuff dippers who keep tobacco between the gums and cheek for prolonged periods of time, the relative risk of developing carcinomas of the gingival or buccal mucosa may increase up to 50 times.[3]

The tracing of carcinogen(s) responsible for the development of oral cancers should not comprise an insurmountable task because of the few items involved. Betel nuts appear to be the main, if not the only source of oral carcinogens in Papua New Guinea, whereas tobacco represents the source of carcinogens among snuff dippers (Table 1). By applying several of the new techniques of analytical chemistry, a virtually complete identification of the chemicals in betel nut, betel leaf, and tobacco is feasible. Once the various components are isolated, the highly sensitive and economic short-term tests for gentoxicity can be applied to detect their mutagenic, clastogenic, and recombinogenic properties.[10,11] The usefulness of these short-term tests is based on a fairly good correlation between mutagenicity of a compound and its carcinogenicity in various rodent species.[12,13] There is a general agreement that chemicals which are positive in several genotoxicity tests are likely to be carcinogenic for various animals and should be placed on a list of probable human carcinogens.

Oral carcinogenesis among betel quid and tobacco chewers also offers the unique opportunity to test the value of various short-term assays in predicting risks for cancer in man. For example, bioassays for clastogenicity, mutagenicity, and gene conversion can be readily applied to the saliva of "pan", betel nut, and tobacco chewers.[14] The micronucleus test can be used on smears of the buccal mucosa, which is the main target tissue of the carcinogenic agents in the case of tobacco and betel nut chewers.[15] The simplicity of these short-term bioassays permits the screening of larger population segments at high or low risk for oral and esophageal cancer. It is this application of newer chemical procedures in combination with a battery of genotoxicity tests which may lead to a more profound understanding of the etiology of cancers of the upper alimentary tract.

Table 1
VARIATIONS IN THE HABIT OF CHEWING BETEL NUT AND TOBACCO

Betel nut and tobacco combinations	Geographic locations
Fresh betel nut + lime	Papua, New Guinea
Fresh betel nut + lime + betel leaf	Assam, Meghalaya, Nagaland, Manipur, Mizoram, Hills of Kerala
Dried betel nut slices + lime + betel leaf + tobacco (several types)	Mainly the northern states of India
Pretreated betel nut + lime + betel leaf + tobacco (several types)	Mainly the southern states of India, Sri Lanka, Malaysia, South Pacific Islands
Pretreated betel nut + lime + betel leaf + tobacco + plant seeds + perfume + catechin	Mainly the southern states of India, Sri Lanka, Malaysia, South Pacific Islands
Tobacco + lime + wood ash (nass)	Iran, Soviet Union
Tobacco + lime (khaini)	Bihar
Tobacco (chewing tobacco)	Worldwide
Tobacco (snuff dipping)	South Carolina

II. VARIATIONS IN CHEWING HABITS

Undoubtedly, the number of items and chemicals involved in oral carcinogenesis of betel nut users or tobacco chewers is considerably smaller than the multitude of compounds in the complex diets of population groups at high or low risk for stomach or colon cancers. Moreover, the variations in chewing habits and in the preparation of pans are limited. Thus, a virtually complete assessment of the exposure of the oral mucosa to carcinogenic, co-carcinogenic, and anticarcinogenic agents of a pan should be feasible. Nevertheless, there are local variations in the composition of the ''pan''. A few of them, as encountered in various geographic regions and among various population groups, are summarized in Table 1.

It is conceivable that the site of carcinogenesis is influenced not only by the type of carcinogenic or co-carcinogenic ingredients of a quid but also by the manner of chewing. For example, population groups differ greatly in their frequencies of spitting or swallowing during a chewing period. The particular chewing habit among the various tribes of the northeastern region of India (e.g., Assam, Meghalaya, Nagaland, Mainpuri) is a good example of one extreme case. For example, the Khasis of Meghalaya usually chew one quarter of a fresh or dry betel nut and part of a lime-covered betel leaf. As a rule, the inclusion of chewing tobacco (with the exception of some females), spices or perfumes is avoided. Thus, this unique situation favors an investigation into the length of exposure of the oral and esophageal mucosa to chemicals which are released from the betel nut and leaf during the course of a day. The number of chewing periods is shown in Figure 1. The population segment examined included villagers, bazaar salesmen, university students, and clerical staff. If we assume an average of 12 min per chewing period, then the oral mucosa is exposed daily for about 3.5 hr to chemicals released from betel nut and betel leaf (see also Section V). Among betel nut chewers of 35 years of age and older, the frequency of oral carcinomas rises significantly. The average age of onset of chewing among Khasis was about 12 years. Thus, in the period between onset of chewing and diagnosis of tumors, the oral mucosa was exposed for about 28,000 hr (equal to roughly 3.2 years of continuous chewing) to betel nut and betel leaf extracts. Danish snuff chewers keep the tobacco in their mouth for about 15.7 hr per day, which amounts to a life mean exposure time of 196,632 hr (equivalent to about 22 years),[16] and Swedish schoolchildren aged 13 to 14 years hold the snuff for an average of 3.5 hr per day.[17] It appears likely, albeit unproven, that during these long exposure periods the oral mucosa will be exposed to initiating as well as to promoting agents. Lime, which irritates the mucosa and leads to hyperplasia, could act as a promoting factor. The calculations of exposure times suffer from one fault. They do not

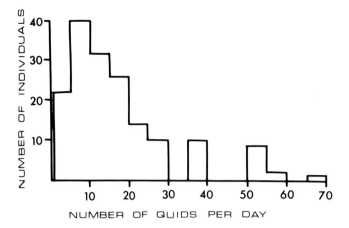

FIGURE 1.   Frequency distribution of the number of quids (betel nut, betel leaf and lime) consumed per day among Khasis of Meghalaya (India).

reveal the period required to initiate carcinogenesis. The initiation time may conceivably comprise only a single fraction of the entire chewing period. Thus, chewing betel quids for 12 years or snuff for 22 years may not be required for the induction of oral carcinomas.

III. MUTAGENS AND CARCINOGENS IN BETEL QUID AND ITS COMPONENTS

The short-term tests for genotoxicity can be used to trace compounds with mutagenic/ clastogenic, and by impliation, carcinogenic properties. These tests are usually applied at first to crude extracts and thereafter to different fractions separated by thin-layer, gel, gas or high pressure liquid chromatography, and finally to purified chemicals. Ideally, tests for carcinogenic properties should be performed in parallel to the genotoxicity studies. However, the enormous cost of the rodent tests for carcinogenicity excludes such an approach. The more realistic way is to examine the isolated compounds with a battery of short-term genotoxicity assays and to use the results to construct a priority list for future carcinogenicity tests on rodents. Currently we are applying this approach in the detection of hazardous compounds in betel nut and betel leaf.

Preliminary studies in our laboratories have shown that the tannic acid fraction derived from betel nuts possesses appreciable genotoxic activity. Tannic acid-containing fractions can induce chromatid breaks and exchanges in mammalian cells (Table 2) and gene conversion in yeast. These results agree with the observation that tannic acids of other plants are potent genotoxic agents.[18] In an effort to isolate the mutagenic agent(s) from the plant material, extracts of betel nut were subjected to a series of extraction and fractionation procedures routinely used in the study of flavonoid and related polyphenolic compounds.[19] Ground, defatted betel nuts were extracted exhaustively with methanol and the extract reduced to dryness. This residue was taken up into hot water and filtered. The aqueous extract, along with some solid material that precipitated on cooling, was extracted with ethyl acetate and then with n-butanol. Tests for clastogenicity were then run for the ethyl acetate-soluble material, the n-butanol-soluble material, and the aqueous material left after extraction. Results from these tests are shown in Table 2.

The ethyl acetate-soluble fraction was subjected to column chromatography on Sephadex® LH-20 using acetone-water mixture as the developing solvents. Results of the column procedure are shown in Figure 2. A major constituent of this fraction appears to be the (+)-catechin (Figure 4, Structure I). The presence of (+)-catechin in betel nut was previously reported by Govindarajan and Mathew.[20,21] (+)-Catechin displays a strong mutagenic ac-

Table 2
CHROMOSOME ABERRATIONS INDUCED BY VARIOUS BETEL NUT FRACTIONS

% Metaphases with chromosome aberrations (no. of aberrations/cell) in betel nut fractions

Dilution	Ethyl acetate		n-Butanol		H₂O after extraction	
	− Mn	+ Mn	− Mn	+ Mn	− Mn	+ Mn
1:8	39.3(1.1)	T[a]	T	T	T	T
1:16	7.4	T	T	T	T	T
1:32	0.6	T	T	T	37.4(1.3)	T
1:64		50.0(5.3)	MI[b]	T		T
1:128	0.5		21.6(0.25)	T		61.9(4.1)
1:256	0.5	6.3	10.0	MI	0.5	22.0
1:512	0.4	0.3	2.8	55.5(8.2)	0.3	3.5

[a] T = toxic.
[b] MI = mitotic inhibition.

tivity, as shown in Table 3. The existence of other similar compounds in the ethyl acetate-soluble fraction is suggested by the chromatographic characteristics and color reactions of several of the spots. Efforts to isolate these components are underway.

Resolution of the *n*-butanol-soluble materials presents a greater difficulty using the above methods. Color reactions and solubility characteristics suggest the presence of complex, possibly polymeric, phenolic compounds in this fraction. Such compounds have been reported in betel nut by numerous workers.[20-23] At the time of this writing, work is being directed toward developing chromatographic systems capable of resolving the complex mixture.

Apart from phenolics, the betel nut contains the alkaloids arecoline, its hydrolyzed product arecaidine, guvacine, and guvacoline.[24] The role of the alkaloids in the development of oral or esophageal carcinomas is difficult to assess. Arecoline and arecaidine showed transforming[25] and clastogenic[26,27] properties.

The betel quid consists of betel nut plus a variety of other substances wrapped in a leaf of *Piper betle,* a species belonging to the black pepper family, *Piperaceae.* In order to arrive at a fuller understanding of the mutagenic and carcinogenic activities of a total quid, it is necessary to know what compounds are contributed by the wrapper leaf. We have therefore undertaken a study of phenolic compounds of *P. betle* leaves. The procedures are described by Wilkins and Bohm.[19] Figure 3 shows a two-dimensional chromatogram of the *P. betle* leaf flavonoids plus related polyphenolic compounds. Flavonoids of *P. betle* are C-glycosylated flavones based upon apigenin (Figure 4, Structure II) and luteolin (Figure 4, Structure III) in Figure 4. Establishment of total structures awaits isolation of sufficient material for proton magnetic resonance spectroscopy. Nonflavonoid components of the leaf, marked by "b" on the diagram, comprise a group of low molecular weight phenolic compounds whose structures will also be studied.

Another ingredient of a quid "pan" or "nass" is tobacco, which demands particular attention. The carcinogenicity of "nass", which consists of tobacco and lime only, is beyond any doubt.[28] Most pans in India contain relatively large quantities of tobacco, which could be involved in the induction of oral and esophageal carcinomas. The amount of tobacco chewed and swallowed daily is by no means negligible. A discourse on the chemistry of tobacco leaves would be beyond the aim of this short review. It may suffice to state that extracts of Indian tobacco widely used in pans are genotoxic,[29] that several *N*-nitrosamines of tobacco are potent carcinogens,[30-33] and that many clastogens can be found among the large groups of phenolics uncovered in tobacco leaves.[18,34-35]

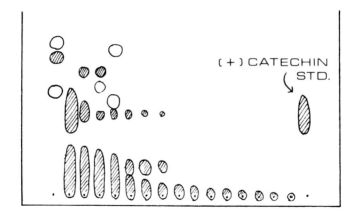

FIGURE 2.   Ethyl acetate-soluble material. LH-20 column fractions. (+)Ca-
techin used as standard marker. Lined spots gave color reactions characteristic
of catechin-like flavonoids. Chromatographic conditions: Polyamid DC6.6
using benzene-methylethyl ketone-methanol-formic acid.

To complicate matters, a betel quid contains various seeds, including anise *(Pimpinella anisum)* and fennel *(Foeniculum vulgare)*. These seeds contain an array of chemicals,[36] some of which (e.g., quercetin) are definitely genotoxic.

The chemical analyses combined with genotoxicity tests revealed mutagens, clastogens, and gene convertants in all the examined ingredients of a pan. Which of them will prove to be carcinogenic in animal experiments remains to be determined. Neither do we know which of these compounds are involved in the etiology of cancers of the oral cavity, pharynx, and esophagus of pan chewers. All hitherto performed rodent tests have uncovered the carcinogenic capacity of betel nut[37-39] and tobacco[40] extracts, but did not point to any single compound as the main carcinogen.

The tracing of the chemicals involved in the etiology of pan-induced cancer is fraught with difficulties. This task is particularly aggravated by an apparently unlimited number of ways of preparing individual pan ingredients. Betel nuts are cured using various ingredients, including "Chogoru", and barks of *Eugenia sambulana, Pterocarpus santalinus, Ficus religiosa,* etc.[23] The used tobacco can be dried, fermented, or perfumed. An examination of tobacco leaves purchased at several bazaars in Shillong (Meghalaya, India) revealed the presence of at least two mold species, which were identified as *Penicillium implicatum* Biourge and *P. decumbens* Thom.[63] The levels of mycotoxins in pan ingredients are unknown, although mold infections may be quite prevalent during the wet seasons.

Another Herculean task is the unraveling of all possible interactions between pan components which may inhibit or enhance carcinogenicity. For example, aqueous betel leaf extracts completely suppressed the carcinogenic activity of betel nut extracts when injected concurrently into rats.[39] On the other hand, rats on a betel leaf diet developed epidermal hyperplasia of the esophagus and forestomach.[41] The precise role of lime in the development of oral cancers also remains a mystery. Undoubtedly, it causes an irritation of the mucosa. When applied to the cheek pouch of hamsters, a series of anomalies, including hyperplasia, hyperkeratosis, and cellular atypia, result.[42] However, lime could conceivably act by elevating the pH,[43] which in turn may affect the metabolism of phenolics, including the tannin (unpublished results). Other possible actions of lime could include alteration of arecoline[44,45] and the release of aromatic oils from the areca nut.[46]

IV. MUTAGENS IN THE SALIVA OF BETEL QUID CHEWERS

The chewing of betel nuts, tobacco, betel leaves, and various seeds of a pan releases numerous chemicals into the saliva. It appears likely that saliva-borne mutagens and car-

Table 3
CLASTOGENICITY OF BETEL NUT FRACTIONS AND COMPOUNDS

	Chromosome aberrations in CHO cells			
Extracts	**Dilution**	**− Mn**	**Dilution**	**+ Mn**
Betel nut *(Areca catechu)*				
Ethyl acetate extract	1:8	39.3	1:64	50.0
Butanol extract	1:128	21.6	1:512	55.5
H_2O after extraction	1:32	37.4	1:128	61.9
Betel leaf *(Piper betle)*				
Ethyl acetate extract	1:2	1.2	1:2	33.3
Butanol extract	1:64	33.3	—	—
H_2O extract	1:8	12.3	—	—

	Chromosome aberrations in CHO cells			
Chemical	**Concentration (mg/mℓ)**	**− Mn**	**Concentration (mg/mℓ)**	**+ Mn**
Delphinidin	0.28	5.0	0.28	84.6
(+)Catechin	0.60	6.1	0.15	51.7
Cyanidin	0.40	4.8	0.40	48.4
"Tannic acid"	0.15	46.2	0.02	40.0
Arecoline	0.40	13.9	—	—

cinogens can then affect the mucosal tissues of the oral cavity, pharynx and, on swallowing, the mucosa of the esophagus. To test this assumption, we examined the level of genotoxic activity found in the saliva of volunteers who chewed either a complete pan or its various components.

The saliva of eight nonchewing, nonsmoking individuals (22 to 42 years of age) lacked genotoxic activity, as determined by the chromosome aberration test on Chinese hamster ovary (CHO) cells, mutation assays in *Salmonella typhimurium*, or the gene conversion test in the D7 strain of yeast. After a few minutes (3 to 10 min) of actively chewing a pan, dried betel nut slices, cured betel nut pieces, betel leaf, Pan Bahar, or perfumed Indian tobacco (Sapuri), respectively, the saliva samples of the volunteers showed relatively potent clastogenic activities.[14] Chromatid breaks, single and multiple chromatid exchanges, and acentric fragments were seen on the first metaphase plates following exposure to the saliva samples of the chewers of pan or its ingredients (Figures 5 and 6). On subsequent metaphase plates, a relatively high percentage of ring chromosomes and dicentrics was observed. One or more micronuclei occurred in 32 to 55% of all examined CHO cells which were exposed for 3 hr to the saliva of pan, betel nut, or Indian tobacco chewers and sampled two days after exposure (Figures 7 and 8). After removal of the pan and its various components, the chromosome-damaging capacity of the saliva rapidly disappeared (Figures 9 and 10). Removal of the pan from the mouth of volunteers simulates the behavior of chewers who spit during their chewing period. The results indicate that relatively high levels of clastogenic activities are only present in the saliva during the actual chewing period.[14] Comparable results were obtained by using another genotoxicity assay, namely, the induction of gene conversion in the D7 strain of yeast (Table 4).

The complexity of the mutagenic load of the saliva of quid users becomes evident from the observation that the chewing of betel nut, betel leaf, Indian tobacco, as well as a mixture of seeds resulted in the appearance of a clastogenic activity. Obviously, several different genotoxic agents must be released into the saliva of pan chewers. This conclusion is in agreement with the observation that various extracts of betel nut (Table 2), betel leaf,[47] and

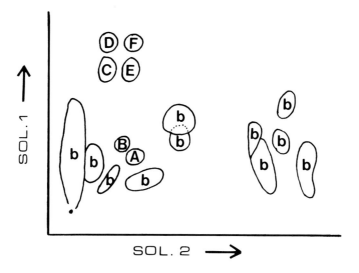

FIGURE 3.   2D Chromatogram of *Piper betle* flavonoids and related phenolics. Spots A, B, C, D, E, and F are C-glycosylflavones; spots marked ''b''
are nonflavonoid. Chromatographic conditions: Polyamide DC6.6 using water-
n-butanol-acetone-dioxane as solvent 1 and benzene-methylethyl ketone-meth-
anol-water as solvent 2.

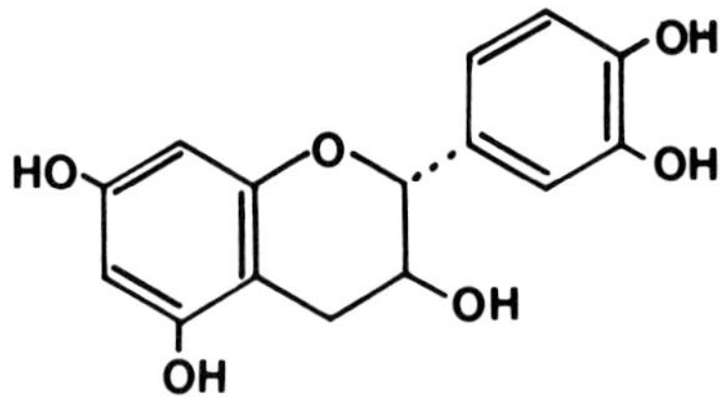

I (+)-CATECHIN

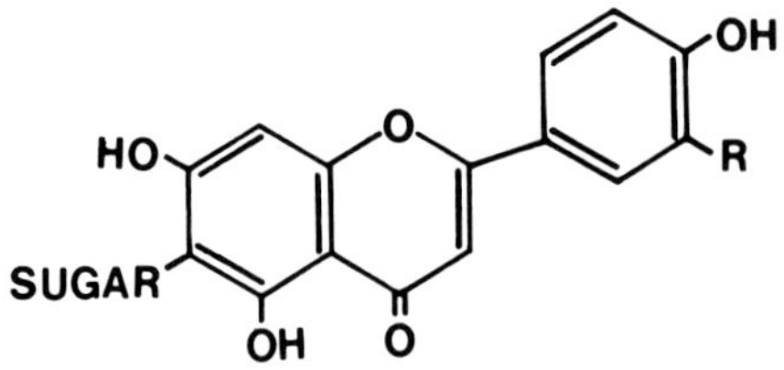

II R = H   6-C-GLYCOSYLAPIGENIN (Spots E, F in
                                    Figure 3)

III R = OH   6-C-GLYCOSYLLUTEOLIN (Spots A, B, C,
                                      and D in Figure 3)

FIGURE 4.   Molecular structure of betel nut and betel leaf compounds.

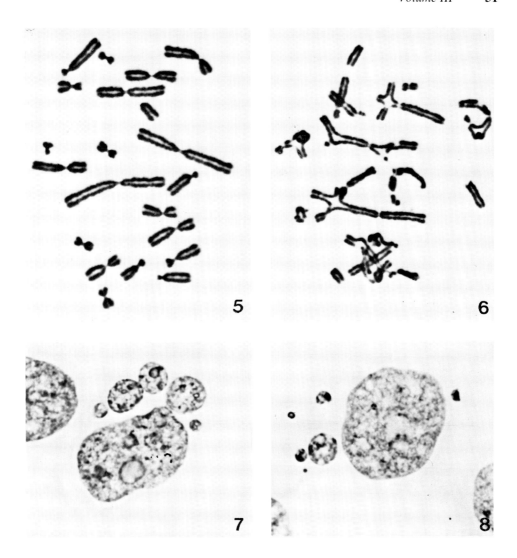

FIGURE 5.   Lack of chromosome aberrations in a CHO cell exposed to saliva of a nonsmoking, nonchewing (betel quid) individual. FIGURE 6. Several chromatid breaks and exchanges in a CHO cell exposed for 3 hr to saliva of a betel quid-chewing individual. FIGURE 7. Micronuclei in CHO cells sampled 48 hr after a 3 hr exposure to saliva of a volunteer chewing Indian tobacco. FIGURE 8. Micronuclei in CHO cells sampled 48 hr after a 3 hr exposure to betel nut pieces (Supari).

Indian Jaffua tobacco[29] are positive in one or the other in vitro assay for genotoxicity. The multitude of mutagenic, and by implication carcinogenic agents also becomes evident when different compounds are isolated from betel nuts, leaves, and tobacco and individually tested for their mutagenic properties (Table 3).

V. TANNIC ACID IN THE SALIVA OF A POPULATION OF BETEL NUT USERS

Tests for mutagens, recombinogens, and clastogens require the sterile, temperature-controlled conditions of a research laboratory. They cannot be readily applied to screen larger population groups under ''field conditions''. We therefore searched for simpler methods

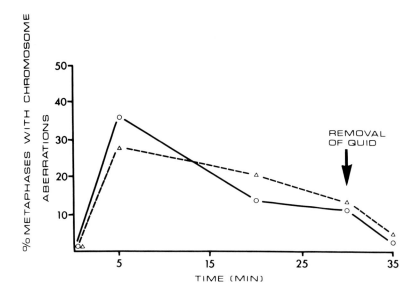

FIGURE 9.   Frequency of metaphase plates with chromosome aberrations in CHO cells exposed to saliva collected from two volunteers during and after chewing a total betel quid. The quid was removed from the mouth after a 30 min chewing period (arrow).

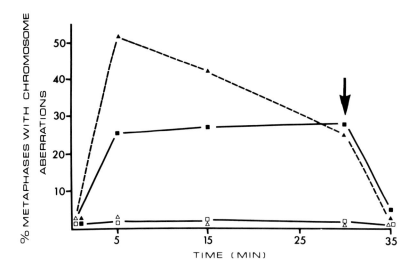

FIGURE 10.   Frequency of metaphase plates with chromosome aberrations in CHO cells exposed to saliva collected from two volunteers during and after chewing a Pan Bahar mixture. The Pan Bahar was removed from the mouth after a 30 min chewing period (arrow).

which may provide information as to the amount of mutagens or carcinogens released from the betel nut into the saliva of chewers. The quantitation of "tannic acid" in the saliva appeared suitable for this purpose. First, the largest proportion of mutagenic activity of betel nut extracts was found in the tannic acid-containing fraction. Second, the sensitive but simple vanillin-HCl procedure of detecting tannins[48] can be readily used on saliva samples. Third, collected saliva samples can be preserved and stored for later analysis of the tannins. However, the vanillin test is positive with a great variety of tannins at different stages of polymerization. Thus the test results give an overview of tannins rather than information on one particular chemically defined compound.

Table 4
INDUCTION OF GENE CONVERSION IN YEAST BY SALIVA OF
VOLUNTEERS CHEWING PAN BAHAR OR BETEL LEAVES

		Convertants/10^5 survivors[a]		
Sample	Mn^{++} ($10^{-4}M$)	Before chewing	During chewing	After chewing
Pan Bahar	$-Mn^{++}$	2.7	6.7	2.6
	$+Mn^{++}$	2.5	15.6	3.7
Betel leaves	$-Mn^{++}$	3.0	3.3	2.9
	$+Mn^{++}$	2.6	3.2	3.0

[a]   *Saccharomyces cerevisiae* strain D7; spontaneous frequency is 2.7 convertants per 10^5 survivors.

Table 5
RELEASE OF "TANNIC ACIDS" INTO THE
SALIVA OF KHASIS CHEWING ONE
QUARTER OF BETEL NUT AND BETEL
LEAF WITH LIME

	Tannic acid/cc saliva			
	Prior to chewing	Chewing (min)		
Individual chewing pattern		3	15	25
Vigorous chewing	6	720	19	4
Vigorous chewing	0	1280	21	22
Chewing	11	105	2080	28
Slow chewing	0	65	28	30

The first question we asked concerned the appearance and survival of tannins in the saliva of betel nut chewers. The study was restricted to Khasis (Meghalaya, India) who chew, as a rule, one quarter of a raw betel nut and part of a betel leaf containing various amounts of lime. Variations in the appearance and disappearance of tannins from the saliva of chewers are shown in Table 5. The observed differences among individuals seem to be mainly due to different chewing patterns. Older persons lacking most of their teeth are unable to crush the relatively hard betel nut pieces. This "sucking" rather than biting of the betel nut releases only relatively small amounts of tannic acids into the saliva. On the other hand, a vigorous biting of the nut seems to favor a release of tannins detectable by the vanillin-HCl procedure. Spitting, which is widespread among southern Indian pan chewers, is virtually unknown among the Khasis. Thus entire chewed nuts and leaves are swallowed. Only 4 out of 125 Khasis interviewed admitted to occasional spitting. Depending on the speed of grinding up the betel nut within the mouth and the time of swallowing the nut fragments, the tannic acid levels peak within 3 to 15 min and then rapidly decline. These results, combined with the information about the number of quids chewed per day, permit us to calculate the time that the mucosa of the oral cavity is exposed to genotoxic agents released from betel nut and betel leaves.

VI. INTERACTION BETWEEN BETEL QUID COMPONENTS

The genotoxicity of complex mixtures is difficult to assess. The mutagenic, clastogenic, and recombinogenic actions of a mixture of compounds are rarely a simple product of the genotoxic activity of each individual component. Reactions between chemicals can enhance

Table 6
ENHANCED CLASTOGENIC ACTIVITY FOLLOWING CONCURRENT APPLICATION OF CHEMICALS FOUND IN A BETEL QUID

Chromosome aberrations[a]

	—	Quercetin (100 μg/mℓ)	Chlorogenic acid (200 μg/mℓ)	Eugenol (200 μg/mℓ)	Chlorogenic acid (25 μg/mℓ) plus Mn^{++} ($10^{-4}M$)
Arecoline (400 μg/mℓ)	13.9(0.23)	92.3(6.45)	53.1(4.53)	75.0(8.74)	61.2(8.80)
—		6.2(0.04)	0.9(0.00)	2.0(0.02)	—

[a]   The frequency of chromosome aberrations is expressed as the percentage of metaphase plates with at least one chromatid break and one chromatid exchange, and the average number of chromatid breaks and exchanges per cell (figures in parentheses).

or suppress the genotoxicity of a mixture.[49-52] Furthermore, cellular activation systems can be influenced by plant products (e.g., flavonoids and flavones), leading to enhanced activation or inhibition of benzo[a]pyrene or aflatoxin B_1.[53] The concurrent application of benzo[a]pyrene can saturate the metabolic activation system, thus preventing the conversion of benzo[a]pyrene into the ultimate mutagenic form.[54] There can be direct interactions between chemicals, such as are exemplified by the destruction of MNNG through cysteine, which result in a loss of genotoxic activity.[55] Furthermore, one compound could conceivably affect the sensitivity of the target cell toward a second mutagen by affecting the DNA repair systems. Our current understanding of the mechanism used by an organism to handle the influx of thousands of mutagenic and carcinogenic agents is indeed dismal.

Considering that an array of mutagenic and nonmutagenic agents are released from the pan into the saliva and that the saliva by itself contains numerous compounds, one must expect a large number of chemical interactions to occur during a chewing period. However, to study all the possible interactions is technically impossible. The number of permutations rapidly increases with the number of individual compounds. The number of cumulative permutations is 325 for 5, 9864 for 10, and about 6.5×10^{18} for 20 chemicals. Thus, an examination of the genotoxicities of five or more interacting compounds would tax the manpower, culture facilities, and budgets of even the largest laboratories. Our studies on the potentiation effects were restricted to components of betel quids which were added to CHO cells in pairs.[26] The chosen compounds included the alkaloid arecoline from the betel nut (*Areca catechu* L.), eugenol from the betel vine (*Piper betle* L.), chlorogenic acid from tobacco leaves *(Nicotiana tabacum)*, quercetin from fennel seeds (*Foeniculum vulgare* Mill.), and the ubiquitous transition metal Mn^{++}. The clastogenic effects of the concurrent applications of arecoline plus eugenol, arecoline plus quercetin, and arecoline plus chlorogenic acid were greater than the sum of the action of each individual component (Table 6). Similarly, the combinations of arecoline, chlorogenic acid, and Mn^{++} induced frequencies of chromosome aberrations which exceeded the sum of the clastogenic activities of two jointly applied compounds, namely, arecoline plus Mn^{++} or chlorogenic acid plus Mn^{++}.[52]

The above-described interactions between quid components depend on the composition of a pan. Since there are numerous ways to prepare a pan, it would be misleading to assume that all pans will exert the same extent of genotoxicity or carcinogenicity. Alone, various levels of Mn^{++}, Cu^{++}, and Fe^{+++} in the various plant products will greatly alter the genotoxic activity of a pan. Since the content of transition metals is greatly influenced by the composition of the soil, betel nuts and betel leaves grown in different geographical regions may exert different enhancing or inhibiting properties on the genotoxicity of a pan.

Table 7
SALIVA-INDUCED INHIBITION AND ENHANCEMENT OF
CLASTOGENICITY OF BETEL QUID COMPONENTS

Chemicals	Concentration (mg/mℓ)	Chromosome aberrations[a]		
		Chemical alone	Chemical plus complete saliva	Chemical plus de-proteinized saliva
Tannic acid	0.1	62.0(5.6)	3.3(0.2)	56.0(4.1)
Quercetin	0.1	3.0(0.03)	14.3(0.65)	6.9(0.09)
Catechol	0.006	3.3(0.03)	20.0(0.48)	13.8(0.21)

[a] See Table 6 for explanation.

VII. INTERACTION OF BETEL QUID COMPONENTS WITH SALIVA

Since many, if not all, genotoxic agents of a quid will appear in the saliva, the possibility must be explored that their activity could be inhibited or enhanced by saliva components. To yield information on this issue, we examined the action of human saliva on the chromosome-breaking (CHO cells), mutagenic *(S. typhimurium)*, and gene convertogenic (yeast) capacity of compounds found in betel nut, seeds of a pan, and tobacco. The basic experimental design consisted of adding for 3 hr tannic acid, quercetin, or arecoline to CHO cells in the absence or presence of human saliva and examining the frequency of chromosome aberrations 20 hr post-treatment. Complete and deproteinized saliva was used at 25% of the original concentration according to the procedure of Stich et al.[56] The results are shown in Table 7. The different responses of various naturally occurring products to the action of human saliva appear to be of particular interest. The clastogenic activity of the tannic acid fraction of betel nuts was greatly reduced by the complete saliva but remained unaffected by the deproteinized saliva. On the other hand, the clastogenic activity of quercetin and catechol was elevated following incubation with complete as well as with deproteinized saliva.

Human saliva seems to reduce the mutagenic effect of several carcinogenic compounds, including complex mixtures.[57] These results, together with our observation on the inhibition of clastogenic activity of the tannic acid fraction of betel nuts, raise the question as to why the saliva of betel nut chewers showed a strong genotoxic effect.[14] The simplest explanation of this apparently contradictory observation is to assume that the concentration of genotoxic agents in the saliva of betel nut chewers exceeds the level which can be inhibited by saliva. At present, it is unknown whether the inhibitory effect of saliva is simply due to the binding of genotoxic agents or whether more complex enzymatically controlled reactions are involved.

VIII. THE ORAL CAVITY AS A PLACE OF CARCINOGEN AND MUTAGEN ACTIVATION AND INACTIVATION

Mutagens and carcinogens of foods and beverages could conceivably undergo their first changes in the oral cavity. There they could interact with each other as well as with saliva-borne compounds, leading to enhanced or reduced mutagenic or carcinogenic activities. In the case of endogenous nitrosamine formation, the importance of nitrate- and nitrite-carrying saliva has already been recognized.[58-60] Furthermore, we have shown a strong inhibitory action of human saliva on the formation of mutagenic nitrosation products when it is present during nitrosation of methylurea[56] or an extract of salted fish.[61]

Of particular concern should be situations where the mucosa of the oral cavity, pharynx, and esophagus are exposed for prolonged periods to mutagens and/or carcinogens which become released into the saliva during habitual chewing. For example, snuff was kept in the mouth for an average of 5720 hr per year among Danish snuff chewers.[16] Since saliva of snuff dippers contains several nitrosamines,[33] this habit leads to an almost chronic exposure to carcinogens released from tobacco. The Khasis of Meghalaya (India) chew betel nut, betel leaf, and lime for an average total of about 1200 hr per year. Market women, farmers, and workmen, however, may chew betel nut mixtures for over 5000 hr per year. The tribal populations of the northeastern region of India swallow the mutagen- and carcinogen-containing saliva and the chewed betel nut and leaf. This habit must invariably result in an exposure of the mucosa, not only of the oral cavity but also of the esophagus. It could be argued that chewers who predominantly spit may have only a higher risk of cancer of the oral cavity, whereas those who mainly swallow during a chewing period are also at a higher risk for esophageal cancer. The relatively higher frequency of esophageal cancers among the tribes of northeast India and among white-collar workers[62] who tend to swallow the chewed pan ingredients, agrees with such an assumption. In both examples, the saliva would be a carrier of carcinogens which are released from the chewed products. However, many important issues remain unresolved. Can the anticarcinogenic activity of saliva cope with the carcinogens released from a small number of pans or slowly chewed betel quids? To what extent will saliva composition and inactivation capacity vary within a population? What role must one attribute to chemicals released into the saliva by bacteria and dying human cells? Answers to these questions must be sought prior to assessing the effectiveness of protective measures against the health hazard of pan- or nass-containing mutagens.

REFERENCES

1. **Jayant, K., Balakrishnan, V. L., Sanghvi, L. D., and Jussawalla, D. J.,** Quantification of the role of smoking and chewing tobacco in oral, pharyngeal and oesophageal cancer, *Br. J. Cancer,* 35, 232, 1977.
2. **Vogler, W. R., Lloyd, J. W., and Milmore, B. K.,** A retrospective study of etiological factors in cancer of the mouth, pharynx, and larynx, *Cancer,* 15, 246, 1962.
3. **Winn, D. M., Blot, W. J., Shy, C. M., Pickle, L. W., Toledo, M. A., and Fraumeni, J. F., Jr.,** Snuff dipping and oral cancer among women in the Southern United States, *N. Engl. J. Med.,* 304, 745, 1981.
4. **Russell, M. A. H., Jarvis, M. J., and Feyerabend, C.,** A new age for snuff? *Lancet,* 1, 474, 1980.
5. **Hirayama, T.,** Epidemiological evaluation of the role of naturally occurring carcinogens and modulators of carcinogenesis, in *Naturally Occurring Carcinogens-Mutagens and Modulators of Carcinogenesis,* Miller, E. C., Miller, J. A., Hirono, I., Sugimura, T., and Takayama, S., Eds., University Park Press, Baltimore, 1979, 359.
6. **Jussawalla, D. J.,** The problem of cancer in India: an epidemiological assessment, *Gann,* 18, 265, 1976.
7. **Pindborg, J. J., Odont, D., Barnes, D., and Roed-Petersen, B.,** Epidemiology and histology of oral leukoplakia and leukoedema among Papuans and New Guineans, *Cancer,* 22, 379, 1968.
8. **Hirayama, T.,** An epidemiological study of oral and pharyngeal cancer in Central and South-East Asia, *Bull. WHO,* 34, 41, 1966.
9. **Wahi, P. N.,** The epidemiology of oral and oropharyngeal cancer, *Bull. WHO,* 38, 495, 1968.
10. **Stich, H. F. and Acton, A. B.,** Can mutation theories of carcinogenesis set priorities for carcinogen testing programmes? *Can. J. Genet. Cytol.,* 21, 155, 1979.
11. **Stich, H. F. and San, R. H. C., Eds.,** *Short-Term Tests for Chemical Carcinogens,* Springer-Verlag, New York, 1981.
12. **Ames, B. N. and Hooper, N.,** Does carcinogenic potency correlate with mutagenic potency in the Ames assay? *Nature (London),* 274, 19, 1978.
13. **Meselson, M. and Russell, K.,** Comparisons of carcinogenic and mutagenic potency, in *Origins of Human Cancer,* Hiatt, H. H., Watson, J. D., and Winsten, J. A., Eds., Cold Spring Harbor Laboratory, Cold Spring Harbor, N.Y., 1977, 1473.
14. **Stich, H. F. and Stich, W.,** Chromosome-damaging activity of saliva of betel nut and tobacco chewers, *Cancer Lett.,* 15, 193, 1982.

15. **Stich, H. F., Curtis, J. R., and Parida, B. B.,** Application of the micronucleus test to exfoliated cells of high cancer risk groups: tobacco chewers, *Int. J.Cancer,* 30, 553, 1982.
16. **Roed-Petersen, B. and Pindborg, J. J.,** A study of Danish snuff-induced oral leukoplakias, *J. Oral Pathol.,* 2, 301, 1973.
17. **Modéer, T., Lavstedt, S., and Ahlund, C.,** Relation between tobacco consumption and oral health in Swedish schoolchildren, *Acta Odontol. Scand.,* 38, 201, 1980.
18. **Stich, H. F. and Powrie, W. D.,** Plant phenolics as genotoxic agents and as modulators for the mutagenicity of other food components, in *Carcinogens and Mutagens in the Environment, Vol. I, Food Products,* Stich, H. F., Ed., CRC Press, Boca Raton, Fla., 1982.
19. **Wilkins, C. K. and Bohm, B. A.,** Flavonoids of *Heuchera micrantha* var. *Diversifolia, Can. J. Bot.,* 54, 2133, 1976.
20. **Govindarajan, V. S. and Mathew, A. G.,** Polyphenolic substances of areca nut. I. Chromatographic analysis of fresh mature nut, *Phytochemistry,* 2, 321, 1963.
21. **Mathew, A. G. and Govindarajan, V. S.,** Polyphenolic substances of areca nut. II. Changes during maturation and ripening, *Phytochemistry,* 3, 657, 1964.
22. **Mathew, A. G., Parpia, H. A. B., and Govindarajan, V. S.,** The nature of the complex proanthrocyanidins, *Phytochemistry,* 8, 1543, 1969.
23. **Arjungi, K. N.,** Areca nut. A review, *Arzneim. Forsch.,* 26, 951, 1976.
24. **Henry, T. H.,** *Te Plant Alkaloids,* London, 1949.
25. **Ashby, J., Styles, J. A., and Boyland, E.,** Betel nuts, arecaidine, and oral cancer, *Lancet,* 1, 112, 1979.
26. **Stich, H. F., Stich, W., and Lam, P. P. S.,** Potentiation of genotoxicity by concurrent application of compounds found in betel quid: arecoline, eugenol, quercetin, chlorogenic acid and Mn^{++}, *Mutat. Res.,* 90, 355, 1981.
27. **Panigrahi, G. B. and Rao, A. R.,** Chromosome-breaking ability of arecoline, a major betel-nut alkaloid, in mouse bone-marrow cells *in vivo, Mutat. Res.,* 103, 197, 1982.
28. **Paches, A. I. and Milievskaya, I. L.,** Epidemiological study of cancer of the mucous membrane of the oral cavity in the USSR, *Natl. Inst. Health,* 80, 177, 1980.
29. **Umezawa, K., Fujie, S., Sawamura, M., Matsushima, T., Katoh, Y., Tanaka, M., and Takayama, S.,** Morphological transformation, sister chromatid exchanges and mutagenesis assay of betel constituents, *Toxicol. Lett.,* 8, 17, 1981.
30. **Hoffman, D., Adams, J. D., Brunnemann, K. D., and Hecht, S. S.,** Assessment of tobacco-specific N-nitrosamines in tobacco products, *Cancer Res.,* 39, 2505, 1979.
31. **Hoffmann, D., Chen, C. B., and Hecht, S. S.,** The role of volatile and nonvolatile N-nitrosamines in tobacco carcinogenesis, in *A Safe Cigarette?* Banbury Report 3, Gori, G. B. and Bock, F. G., Eds., Cold Spring Harbor Laboratory, Cold Spring Harbor, N.Y., 1980, 113.
32. **Hoffmann, D. and Adams, J. D.,** Carcinogenic tobacco-specific N-nitrosamines in snuff and in the saliva of snuff dippers, *Cancer Res.,* 41, 4305, 1981.
33. **Bhide, S. V., Pratap, A. I., and Shivapurkar, N. M.,** Detection of nitrosamines in a commonly used chewing tobacco, *Food Cosmet. Toxicol.,* 19, 481, 1981.
34. **Snook, M. E., Fortson, P. J., and Chortyk, O. T.,** Gel chromatography for the isolation of phenolic acids from tobacco leaf, *Anal. Chem.,* 53, 374, 1981.
35. **Stich, H. F., Rosin, M. P., Wu, C. H., and Powrie, W. D.,** The action of transition metals on the genotoxicity of simple phenols, phenolic acids and cinnamic acids, *Cancer Lett.,* 14, 251, 1981.
36. **Kunzemann, J. and Herrmann, K.,** Isolierung und Identifizierung der Flavon(ol)-O-glykoside in Kümmel (*Carum carvi* L.), Fenchel (*Foeniculum vulgare* Mill.), Anis (*Pimpinella anisum* L.) und Koriander (*Coriandrum sativum* L.) und von Flavon-C-glykosiden im Anis, *Z. Lebensm. Unters. Forsch.,* 164, 194, 1977.
37. **Bhide, S. V., Shivapurkar, N. M., Gothoskar, S. V., and Ranadive, K. J.,** Carcinogenicity of betel quid ingredients: feeding mice with aqueous extracts and the polyphenol fraction of betel nut, *Br. J. Cancer,* 40, 922, 1979.
38. **Ranadive, K. J., Ranadive, S. N., Shivapurkar, N. M., and Gothoskar, S. V.,** Betel quid chewing and oral cancer: experimental studies on hamsters, *Int. J. Cancer,* 24, 835, 1979.
39. **Shivapurkar, N. M., Ranadive, S. N., Gothoskar, S. V., Bhide, S. V., and Ranadive, K. J.,** Tumorigenic effect of aqueous and polyphenolic fractions of betel nut in Swiss strain mice, *Ind. J. Exp. Biol.,* 18, 1159, 1980.
40. **Umezawa, K., Takayama, S., Fujie, S., Matsushima, T., and Sugimura, T.,** *In vitro* transformation of hamster embryo cells by betel tobacco extracts, *Toxicol. Lett.,* 2, 243, 1978.
41. **Mori, H., Matsubara, N., Ushimaru, Y., and Hirono, I.,** Carcinogenicity examination of betel nuts and *Piper* betel leaves, *Experientia,* 35, 384, 1979.
42. **Dunham, L. J., Muir, C. S., and Hamner, J. E., III,** Epithelial atypia in hamster cheek pouches treated repeatedly with calcium hydroxide, *Br. J. Cancer,* 20, 588, 1966.
43. **Malhotra, S. L.,** New approaches to the causation and prevention of cancer of epithelial surfaces, *Med. Hypoth.,* 2, 279, 1977.

44. **Boyland, E. and Nery, R.,** Mercapturic acid formation during the metabolism of arecoline and arecaidine in the rat, *Biochem. J.,* 113, 123, 1969.

45. **Nieschulz, O. and Schmersahl, P.,** Zur Pharmakologie der Wirkstoffe des Betel, *Arzneim. Forsch.,* 18, 222, 1968.

46. **Steinegger, E. and Häusel, R.,** *Lehrbuch der Allgemeinen Pharmakognosie,* Springer-Verlag, Berlin, 1963.

47. **Sadasivan, G., Rani, G., and Kumari, C. K.,** Chromosome-damaging effect of betel leaf, *Mutat. Res.,* 57, 183, 1978.

48. **Broadhurst, R. B. and Jones, W. T.,** Analysis of condensed tannins using acidified vanillin, *J. Sci. Food Agric.,* 29, 788, 1978.

49. **Stich, H. F., Wei, L., and Whiting, R. F.,** Enhancement of the chromosome-damaging action of ascorbate by transition metals, *Cancer Res.,* 39, 4145, 1979.

50. **Rosin, M. P. and Stich, H. F.,** Assessment of the use of the *Salmonella* mutagenesis assay to determine the influence of antioxidants on carcinogen-induced mutagenesis, *Int. J. Cancer,* 23, 722, 1979.

51. **Rosin, M. P. and Stich, H. F.,** Inhibitory effect of reducing agents on N-acetoxy- and N-hydroxy-2-acetylaminofluorene-induced mutagenesis, *Cancer Res.,* 38, 1307, 1978.

52. **Rosin, M. P.,** Inhibition of genotoxic activities of complex mixtures by naturally occurring agents, in *Carcinogens and Mutagens in the Environment, Vol. I, Food Products,* Stich, H. F., Ed., CRC Press, Boca Raton, Fla., 1982.

53. **Wattenberg, L. W.,** Naturally occurring inhibitors of chemical carcinogenesis, in *Naturally Occurring Carcinogens-Mutagens and Modulators of Carcinogenesis,* Miller, E. C., Miller, J. A., Hirono, I., Sugimura, T., and Takayama, S., Eds., University Park Press, Baltimore, 1979, 315.

54. **Stich, H. F., Rosin, M. P., Wu, C. H., and Powrie, W. D.,** The use of mutagenicity testing to evaluate food products, in *Mutagenicity: New Horizons in Genetic Toxicology,* Heddle, J. A., Ed., Academic Press, New York, 1982, 117.

55. **Wei, L., Whiting, R. F., and Stich, H. F.,** Inhibition of chemical mutagenesis: an application of chromosome aberration and DNA synthesis assays using cultured mammalian cells, in *Short-Term Tests for Chemical Carcinogens,* Stich, H. F. and San, R. H. C., Eds., Springer-Verlag, New York, 1981, 428.

56. **Stich, H. F., Rosin, M. P., and Bryson, L.,** The inhibitory effect of whole and deproteinized saliva on mutagenicity and clastogenicity resulting from a model nitrosation reaction, *Mutat. Res.,* 97, 283, 1982.

57. **Nishioka, H., Nishi, K., and Kyokane, K.,** Human saliva inactivates mutagenicity of carcinogens, *Mutat. Res.,* 85, 323, 1981.

58. **Walters, C. L., Carr, F. P. A., Dyke, C. S., Saxby, M. J., Smith, P. L. R., and Walker, R.,** Nitrite sources and nitrosamine formation *in vitro* and *in vivo, Food Cosmet. Toxicol.,* 17, 473, 1979.

59. **Tannenbaum, S. R.,** Endogenous formation of nitrite and N-nitroso compounds, in *Naturally Occurring Carcinogens-Mutagens and Modulators of Carcinogenesis,* Miller, E. C., Miller, J. A., Hirono, I., Sugimura, T., and Takayama, S., Eds., University Park Press, Baltimore, 1979, 211.

60. **Tannenbaum, S. R., Archer, M. C., Wishnok, J. S., and Bishop, W. W.,** Nitrosamine formation in human saliva, *J. Natl. Cancer Inst.,* 60, 251, 1978.

61. **Stich, H. F., Chan, P. K. L., and Rosin, M. P.,** Inhibitory effects of phenolics on the formation of mutagenic nitrosation products of salted fish, *Int. J. Cancer,* 30, 719, 1982.

62. **Shanta, V. and Krishnamurthi, S.,** Further studies in aetiology of carcinomas of the upper alimentary tract, *Br. J. Cancer,* 17, 8, 1963.

63. **Chakravarty, P.,** Personal communication.

Chapter 6

THE POSSIBLE ROLE OF OPIUM AND TOBACCO PYROLYSATES IN ESOPHAGEAL CANCER

Nicholas E. Day, Christian Malaveille, Marlin Friesen, and Helmut Bartsch

TABLE OF CONTENTS

I. EPIDEMIOLOGICAL EVIDENCE

Localized areas of very high incidence of cancer of the esophagus occur in several of the nonindustrialized areas of the world. It is likely that the environmental carcinogens which are inducing the disease in these areas are either part of the natural environment or result from some cultural modification of substances in the natural environment. We shall discuss the results of investigations in two of these foci of high incidence, northeast Iran and the Transkei (southeast Africa), with particular emphasis on the former. To provide a background, however, it is useful to briefly discuss the results of studies in Western countries where the major risk factors for esophageal cancer have been identified.

A. Role of Tobacco Pyrolysates in Esophageal Cancer

In Western Europe and North America, the major causes of esophageal cancer are alcohol and tobacco.[1,2] The risks associated with these two factors combine multiplicatively, leading to an incidence among heavy consumers of both that is more than 100-fold higher than the incidence among light consumers or abstainers. The use of strong alcoholic drinks appears to be more potent than wine or beer, for a given intake of ethanol.[3] Alcohol itself has never been shown experimentally to have carcinogenic or mutagenic activity, so that its presumed role in the development of esophageal cancer is to potentiate the action of the carcinogens in the tobacco smoke residues.

The most noteworthy feature of the epidemiology of esophageal cancer is the very sharp gradient in incidence seen in several areas of the world, circumscribing areas of outstandingly high incidence.[4-6] Parts of Brittany and Normandy provide an example of such areas in Europe,[7] and there seems little doubt that the high risk in these parts of northwest France is related to local patterns of consumption of alcohol, in particular apple brandy, home distilled or commercial. That is to say that in these areas of France of high incidence, although there is widespread exposure to tobacco smoke residues potentially carcinogenic for the esophagus, the high risk is due mainly to the unusual level of sensitizing or potentiating factors. When turning to the situation in northeast Iran or the Transkei, it must therefore be borne in mind that the powerfully mutagenic substances we describe are probably only one component in a multi-component etiology, and not solely responsible for the very high incidence observed.

The role of tobacco in the etiology of esophageal cancer is particularly interesting in the Transkei, where esophageal cancer is unusually common in the south among both sexes. Unlike Europe and North America, alcohol does not seem to be a major potentiating factor. Inadequate diet and nutrition have been documented[8] related to impoverishment of the soil and rural over-population. The major environmental factor, however, distinguishing the high incidence area of the Transkei from neighboring areas of lower incidence is the use of home grown tobacco,[9] especially pipe smoking,[10] and the use of pipe tobacco residues and smoke condensates. The liquid collecting in the bowl of the pipe, called injonga, is sucked into the mouth through a thin straw, and the tobacco residues in the bowl of the pipe, called isixaxa, are chewed.[11] Use of injonga is more frequent than of isixaxa and is common among both sexes in the areas of the Transkei where esophageal cancer is of high incidence. It is little used in the low incidence areas. Case-control evidence linking use of either injonga or isixaxa to risk for esophageal cancer does not appear to have been documented, but the co-occurrence in the southern Transkei of the habit with the high risk of the cancer is striking.

B. The Role of Opium Pyrolysates in Esophageal Cancer

Parts of the provinces of Gorgan and Gonbad in northeast Iran have an incidence of esophageal cancer higher in both sexes than has been reported anywhere else in the world. To the north, over the border in Soviet Turkmenistan, the incidence is also high, but to the

Table 1
PREVALENCE OF THE PRESENCE OF
MORPHINE METABOLITES IN THE URINE
OF POPULATIONS AT DIFFERING RISK FOR
ESOPHAGEAL CANCER IN NORTHERN IRAN

	Area of high incidence	Area of low incidence
1973 survey[a]		
Adults over 35 years	51%	11%
1978 survey[b]		
Females over 30 years	31%	6%
Males over 30 years	46%	Not available

[a]   See Reference 12.
[b]   See Reference 16.

west, along the Caspian littoral, the frequency of the disease decreases over a distance of a few hundred kilometers by some 30-fold in women, slightly less in men. A wide ranging series of studies was conducted in the area to determine which environmental factors could be inculpated in the causation of the disease, if indeed the disease were environmental in origin. These studies provide a wide range of negative findings.[12,13] Food and water were extensively analyzed for the presence of polycyclic aromatic hydrocarbons (PAH), nitro-samines, nitrate and nitrite (also measured in saliva), and mycotoxins, with no indication of unusually high values. Wheat and flour were examined for microcontaminants and for foreign seeds, and extracts tested for mutagenicity. Surveys and case-control studies inves-tigated tobacco smoking and chewing, drinking, craft industries and other occupations, peculiarities of food preservation and preparation, and other aspects of lifestyle. Dietary deficiencies (riboflavin, vitamins A and C, and animal protein) clearly characterized those at high risk,[14,15] but among the factors which might be considered as potentially having carcinogenic activity, only the use of opium appeared related to disease risk.

In the initial round of studies, morphine metabolites were found in the urine of 50% of both the female and male adult population of the area of highest incidence (Table 1). By contrast very few positive urines were seen in the areas of lower incidence.[12] Further enquiries revealed that opium was used in several ways by large sections of the high incidence population.[11] Crude opium could be smoked or eaten. When smoked, a thick residue forms in the pipe having an appreciable morphine content (5 to 8%). This residue or dross, known locally as sukhteh, is used in several ways. It is taken by people of all ages, including children, to treat most minor ailments, and it is given to infants to help them sleep. It is eaten by addicts, particularly the poorer ones, either alone or mixed with more crude opium, and it is also used with opium in the preparation of a refined product, shireh. Shireh is obtained by boiling opium, or a mixture of opium and sukhteh, with water, usually in a small copper bowl, filtering several times, and then evaporating the filtrate until a gluey consistency is obtained.

Difficulties arose in designing studies to link opium use more firmly on an individual basis to risk for disease. First, its use is illegal except by the small proportion of the population who register as addicts, so that information obtained systematically by questionnaire from the healthy population is valueless. Second, opium use is freely admitted to and very common among those who are seriously ill. Case-control studies or questionnaire surveys on frequency and type of use were therefore pointless. Consideration was given to identifying physiological or biochemical markers of long-term opium use, related perhaps to morphine tolerance, but tolerance develops over months rather than the decades which would be relevant for these

Table 2

**MUTAGENICITY IN *SALMONELLA TYPHIMURIUM*
STRAINS OF VARIOUS SMOKE CONDENSATES OF
TOBACCO GROWN IN TRANSKEI AND FROM OTHER
COMMERCIAL SOURCES**

Test material[a] (no. of samples tested in parentheses)	Mutagenicity[b] (His^+ revertants/mg)		Ref.
	Strain TA98	Strain TA100	
Injonga (3)	40—130	15—25	11
Isixaxa (7)	55—80	20—30	11
Transkei tobacco smoke conden-sate (1)	900	400	27
Commercial pipe smoke conden-sate (1)	500	320	27
Commercial cigarette smoke con-densate (2)	100—150	240	27
Commercial cigarette cigar and pipe smoke condensate (highest and lowest ranges reported in the literature)	50—2000	n.d.[c]	38
			39
			39
			27
			41
			28

[a]   For definition, see text.
[b]   Assays were carried out in the presence of a rat liver activation system; the number of revertants occurring in control assays has been subtracted.
[c]   n.d. = not determined.

purposes and no progress was made in that direction. The civil disturbances in late 1978 before the Iranian revolution led to the abandon of all work in the field, but at that time three lines of investigation were being pursued. First, an attempt to identify metabolites of opium pyrolysates enabling one to identify sukhteh consumption; second, a case-control study on a household basis, since opium use goes closely by household; and third, more extensive population studies to verify and extend the initial, rather limited findings. Preliminary results from these population studies are also given in Table 1.[16] They corroborate the earlier results. If social conditions had permitted, definitive epidemiological evidence might have been provided by a prospective study. In view of the incompleteness of the epidemiological data, the chemical and biological characterization of sukhteh and other pyrolysates of opium constituents become of prime importance.

II. EXPERIMENTAL STUDIES

A. Mutagens/Carcinogens in Tobacco Pyrolysates

The relationship between smoking and cancer of the lung, esophagus, and larynx in humans, based on epidemiology data is generally established.[17-19] Chemical analysis has indicated that tobacco smoke condensate is an extremely complex mixture containing a number of identified carcinogenic aromatic amines, polycyclic hydrocarbons, and *N*-nitroso compounds.[20-22] However, the carcinogenic potential of the crude material is too great to be explained simply in terms of its content of the identified substances belonging to the three classes of carcinogens mentioned above.[23]

The mutagenic activity of tobacco smoke condensate, which requires the presence of a liver activation system, has been amply demonstrated with activities ranging from 50 to 2000 revertants per milligram condensate in *Salmonella typhimurium* TA98 strain (Table 2). Mutagenicity was shown to be strongly influenced by the source of tobacco, its composition, and by parameters related to the pyrolysis process itself. The total nitrogen, protein nitrogen, and soluble nitrogen content of tobacco leaves were all positively and significantly related to an increase in the mutagenic activity of the corresponding smoke condensates, whereas nicotine, nitrate, and soluble sugar content were not important in contributing to the mutagenicity of such condensates.[24] These results are in agreement with the findings that cigarette smoke condensate and the smoke from pyrolyzed protein show equally high mutagenic activities, while pyrolysis of carbohydrates does not result in appreciable mutagenic activity in many combusted products tested.[25]

Pyrolysis of amino acids, e.g., of D-tryptophan, also yields strongly mutagenic compounds recently characterized as nitrogen-containing heterocyclic aromatic compounds containing an exocyclic amino group (for a review, see Reference 26). These results suggest that some of the potent mutagens in cigarette smoke condensate are nitrogen-containing compounds, which may be formed by pyrolysis of proteins and amino acids in tobacco.

In the Transkei, pipe smoking and the use of home-grown tobacco were shown to be the main environmental factors associated with an increased risk of esophageal cancer in both sexes. Of particular interest is the ingestion of the tobacco residues, injonga and isixaxa, described in an earlier section, which appears to be a habit confined principally to the populations at high risk. Smoke condensates from Transkei tobacco (home-grown), in the form of injonga and isixaxa, were found to revert *Salmonella typhimurium* strains TA98 and TA100, with highest activity toward TA98 (Table 2).[11] Later results[27] confirmed these findings, showing that the mutagenicity of Transkei tobacco for *S. typhimurium* strain TA98 exceeded that of commercial pipe and cigarette tobacco condensate (Table 2), and that enhanced mutagenicity is positively correlated to the high nitrogen content of Transkei tobacco.

Since the presence of identified carcinogens/mutagens in tobacco smoke condensate, as well as the carcinogenic and mutagenic activity of the complex mixtures, has been amply demonstrated, and since the mutagenic activity of Transkei tobacco smoke condensate was in the range of activity reported for commercial cigarette, cigar, or pipe smoke condensates, it is likely that ingestion of mutagens present in isixaxa and injonga contribute to the high incidence of esophageal cancer found in both sexes in Transkei.

B. Genotoxic Compounds Produced by Pyrolysis of Opium and Its Alkaloids

The widespread use of opium in a region of northeast Iran, where esophageal cancer is exceedingly common in both men and women, has been described in an earlier section.

Unlike tobacco smoke condensate, the nature and biological activity of the products derived from the pyrolysis of opium and its major alkaloids have not yet been fully elucidated and most of the investigations are still in progress. Some of the results from attempts to characterize these compounds are summarized below.

1. Mutagenic Activity of Sukhteh, Shireh, and Crude Opium Samples

An initial study[11] reported the mutagenic activity of a small number of samples of sukhteh (opium dross) and virtually no activity for crude opium. These results were confirmed in a second study[28] involving 21 samples of sukhteh (methylene chloride extracts) and 6 samples of opium, collected in the Kerman region of Iran in 1978—1979 (Table 3). Extracts of crude (nonpyrolyzed) opium showed no mutagenic activity in *S. typhimurium* strain TA100 and only sporadic, borderline activity in strain TA98. Similarly, the refined product shireh showed no appreciable mutagenic activity (Table 3). All 21 sukhteh samples were mutagenic in both strains, requiring the presence of a rat liver S9 activation system. When the latter was omitted, mutagenicity in the TA98 strain was decreased by 98%. In all samples mutagenicity was high in TA98. The TA98:TA100 mutagenicity ratio ranged from 2.3 to 5.7 (mean 3.0) (Table 3). The positive correlation between the mutagenic activities in TA98 and TA100 strains ($r = 0.987$; $p < 0.001$; $n = 21$) suggests that the mutagenic compounds present in sukhteh differ in concentration from one sample to another but not in structure.

Table 3

**RAT LIVER S9-MEDIATED MUTAGENICITY OF
SUKHTEH AND OPIUM SAMPLES (METHYLENE
CHLORIDE EXTRACTS) IN *SALMONELLA
TYPHIMURIUM* STRAINS TA98 AND TA100**[11,28]

| Test material (CH$_2$Cl$_2$ extract)[b] | Mutagenicity[a] | | |
| | Revertants/mg extract | | TA98:TA100 mutagenicity ratio |
	TA98	TA100	
Sukhteh			
Mean of 21 samples	700	240	3.0
(range)	(70—1540)	(30—500)	(2.3—5.7)
Opium sample no.			
1	57	0	
2	21	0	
3	19	0	
4	0	0	
5	65	0	
6	0	0	
Mean (n = 6)	27	0	
(range)	(0—65)	0	
Shireh sample no.			
1	5	7	
2	2	5	
3	0	7	
4	5	2	
5	10	10	
6	1	5	
Mean (n = 6)	4	6	
(range)	(0—10)	(2—10)	

[a] Specific mutagenicity was calculated from dose-response curves ranging from 0.1 to 0.9 mg of sukhteh extract/plate and from 0.2 to 3.0 mg of opium extract/plate. The number of revertants/plate occurring spontaneously was subtracted prior to calculation of specific mutagenicity.

[b] For definition, see text.

2. Combustion of Opium and Opium Constituents: Effect of Pyrolysis Temperature and Sample Origin on the Mutagenicity of Opium Smoke Condensates

To facilitate characterization of the substances responsible for the mutagenic activity, pyrolysis of opium and opium constituents was carried out in air in the all-glass combustion apparatus shown in Figure 1.

Figure 2B shows the relationship between the mutagenic activity and temperature for a sample of (Indian) opium pyrolyzed at temperatures ranging from 350 to 600°C. The mutagenicity increased with temperature up to 550°C, but below 350°C, only very small quantities of mutagens were produced. Therefore, subsequent investigations were carried out at 450°C, a pyrolysis temperature located at approximately the middle of the ascending parts of the curve shown in Figure 2B and likely to be close to the temperature reached during opium smoking.

To investigate whether the different levels of mutagenic activity found in sukhteh samples (Table 3) were related to differences in sample origin, and hence to differences in opium composition, opium samples obtained from four different geographical regions were pyrolyzed (Table 4). The S9-mediated mutagenicity of the four opium pyrolysates varied over a threefold range, the highest specific activity being obtained with pyrolysates of Turkish

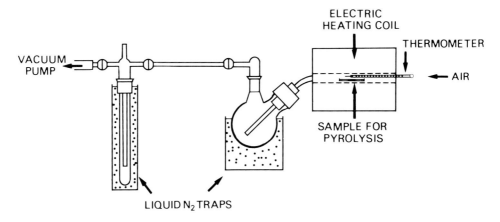

FIGURE 1. Apparatus used to pyrolyze opium and constituents and to collect smoke condensate. Temperatures of 300 to 600°C were produced by an electrical heating coil. Samples of 50 to 100 mg were pyrolyzed in quartz boats. Complete pyrolysis required approximately 30 to 60 sec. Pyrolysis products were drawn out into liquid nitrogen-cooled traps by application of a slight vacuum. After pyrolysis, the residues in the traps were extracted with methylene chloride. The solution was then dried, filtered, and the solvent evaporated at 40°C. Pyrolysis of 100 mg of opium and of 100 mg of morphine yielded about 20 mg and 30 mg of condensates, respectively. (From Malaveille, C. et al., *Carcinogenesis,* 3, 577, 1982. With permission.)

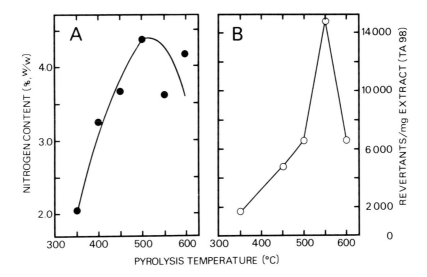

FIGURE 2. (A) Nitrogen content (% w/w) of pyrolyzed Indian opium (methylene chloride extract) as a function of pyrolysis temperature. Each point corresponds to a single determination. (B) S9-mediated mutagenicity in *Salmonella typhimurium* TA98 strain (number of revertants per milligrams of extract) of pyrolyzed Indian opium (methylene chloride extracts) as a function of pyrolysis temperature. (From Malaveille, C. et al., *Carcinogenesis,* 3, 577, 1982. With permission.)

opium and the lowest with Indian opium. Mutagenicity in the presence of a metabolic activation system was 35 to 40 times higher than the direct activity in strain TA98 (Table 4, ratio A:B). Specific mutagenicity of pyrolysates of these opium samples was highest with pyrolyzed Turkish opium and lowest with Indian opium, paralleling the relative concentrations of morphine reported in opium of Turkish (16%) and of Indian (less than 10%) origin.[29]

This similarity in mutagenic behavior, characterized by comparable TA98:TA100 mutagenicity ratios on the one hand, and comparable ratios between direct-acting mutagens and

Table 4

MUTAGENICITY OF PYROLYSIS PRODUCTS (METHYLENE CHLORIDE EXTRACTS) OF OPIUM AND ITS
MAJOR CONSTITUENTS IN *SALMONELLA TYPHIMURIUM* STRAINS TA98 AND TA100

Experiment no.	CH₂Cl₂ extract	Mutagenicity[a] (revertants/mg extract)				TA98:TA100 mutagenicity ratio (A:C)
		TA98		TA100		
		+ S9 A	− S9 B	+ S9 C	− S9 D	
	Pyrolysate of					
1	Morphine	87,500[b](100)	0	50,800[b](100)	1,280	1.7
2	Thebaine	65,500 (75)	400	32,300 (63)	340	2.0
3	Sanguinarine	1,040 (1.2)	550	3,850 (7.6)	2,410	0.3
4	Codeine	1,010 (1.2)	35	590 (1.2)	340	1.7
5	Noscapine	230 (0.3)	0	150 (0.3)	0	1.5
6	Narceine	0 (0)	0	300 (0.6)	100	0
7	Papaverine	70 (0.1)	0	80 (0.2)	0	0.9
8	Cycloartenol	0 (0)	0	0 (0)	0	—
9	β-Sitosterol	0 (0)	0	0 (0)	0	—
	Pyrolysate of opium from					
10	India	5,900	170	2,130	240	2.8
11	Iran	10,100	210	2,320	310	4.4
12	Turkey	17,000	350	5,910	680	2.9
13	Afghanistan	14,400	300	3,730	550	3.9
	Mean (experiments 10—13)	11,900	260	3,520	450	3.5
	(range)	(5,900—17,000)	(170—350)	(2,130—5,910)	(240—680)	(2.8—4.4)
14	Sukhteh (mean) (range[e])	700[c]	15[d]	240[c]	110[d]	3.0
		(70—1,540)	(0—70)	(30—500)	(0—250)	(2.3—5.7)

[a] Mutagenic activity was determined in the presence or absence of fortified rat liver S9. The number of revertants/plate occurring spontaneously was subtracted prior to calculation of specific mutagenicity.

[b] Relative S9-mediated mutagenicity, taking that of morphine pyrolysate as 100.

[c] Rat liver S9-mediated mutagenicity of sukhteh represents the mean of the activities of the 21 samples listed in Table 3.

[d] Direct mutagenicity of sukhteh represents the mean of the activities of the 21 samples measured.

[e] Range of mutagenic activities of the 21 sukhteh samples (Table 3).

From Malaveille, C. et al., *Carcinogenesis*, 3, 577, 1982. With permission.

those requiring metabolic activation on the other, suggests that the mutagenic activities of sukhteh (collected in Iran) and of opium pyrolysate (produced in the laboratory) are due to similar compounds. The 17-times higher S9-mediated mutagenicity of opium pyrolysates as compared with sukhteh may be plausibly explained by more efficient trapping of mutagens in the pyrolysis apparatus (Figure 1) than in the opium pipes from which the sukhteh was collected by scraping off the tarry residues. A differential loss of mutagenic compounds during opium smoking and during subsequent collection of residues may therefore explain the 22-fold range of activities observed for the 21 sukhteh samples tested (Table 3).

A relationship has been noted between the total nitrogen content of tobacco leaf and the mutagenicity of the corresponding tobacco smoke condensate.[24] As nitrogen-containing alkaloids (Figure 3, I—VII) comprise approximately 25% of the weight of crude opium, the relationship between the nitrogen content and the specific mutagenicity of opium pyrolysates was investigated. The results (Figure 2A) revealed a certain parallelism between the nitrogen content of an opium pyrolysate and its specific mutagenicity (Figure 2B). These two variables increased approximately 2- and 7-fold, respectively, when the pyrolysis temperature was raised from 350°C to about 500°C.

The mutagenic activity of major nitrogen-containing opium alkaloids and other constituents (Figure 3, I—IX) was investigated after pyrolysis under conditions identical to those used for crude opium. The results obtained (Table 4) in strains TA98 and TA100 in the presence and absence of rat liver S9 indicate that, after pyrolysis, mutagenic substances are formed from all opium alkaloids. Pyrolyzed plant sterols, such as cycloartenol or β-sitosterol (Figure 3, VII, IX) which do not contain nitrogen, produced little mutagenicity. In general, pyrolysates of all alkaloids required metabolic activation to produce appreciable mutagenicity, and, with the exception of sanguinarine, narceine, and papaverine, the response was higher in strain TA98. When the pyrolysates were compared quantitatively, those of the three alkaloids (morphine, codeine, and thebaine, i.e., those with a phenanthrene-type structure) showed much higher mutagenic activities than the other alkaloids which contained two-membered ring systems only (Figure 3, IV—VI). After pyrolysis, mutagenicity of sangui-

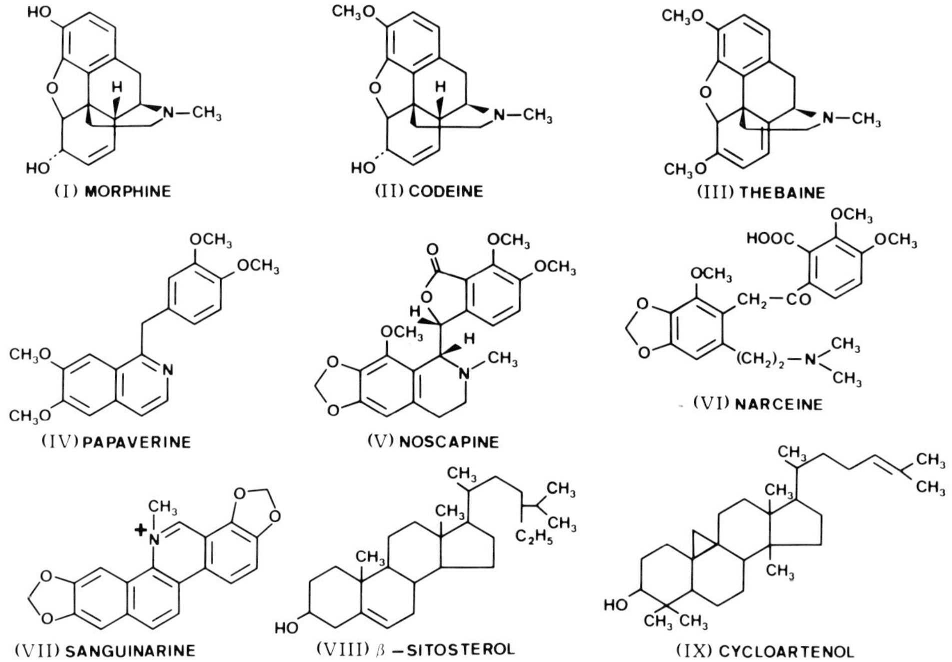

FIGURE 3. Chemical structures of some major alkaloids and plant sterols. (From Malaveille, C. et al., *Carcinogenesis*, 3, 577, 1982. With permission.)

narine (a minor constituent of opium and poppy seed) in TA98 was comparable to that of pyrolyzed codeine, but it behaved differently, as the bacterial mutagen TA98:TA100 ratio was lower and its direct mutagenicity in TA100 strain was appreciable (Table 4).

Of the pyrolysates of the phenanthrene-type alkaloids, those produced from morphine and thebaine were by far the most mutagenic. Despite its structural similarity to morphine, codeine yielded pyrolysis products with only 1% of the mutagenicity of morphine pyrolysate in strain TA98. This points to the importance of the free hydroxyl groups present in morphine, which are probably necessary to produce active mutagens during pyrolysis; mutagenicity decreases drastically when one or two methoxy groups replace the hydroxyl groups in the morphine molecule (see Figure 3, I—III).

The data in Table 5 suggest that the total (S9-mediated) mutagenic activity of opium pyrolysate can be accounted for by the pyrolysis products of the five alkaloids listed. Considering their relative concentration in crude opium and the specific mutagenicity after their pyrolysis, over 84% of the mutagenic activity of (Indian) opium pyrolysate can be attributed to pyrolysis products of morphine and almost 100% to the pyrolysis products of the three phenanthrene type alkaloids.

3. Characterization of Mutagenic Compounds Present in Opium Pyrolysates

Since the mutagenic activity of opium pyrolysates was shown to parallel their nitrogen content (Figure 2), an investigation as to whether primary aromatic amines might be partly responsible for the mutagenicity of opium pyrolysate was conducted. It has been shown that treatment of mutagenic primary aromatic amines with nitrous acid reduces S9-mediated mutagenicity through conversion of the amino into a hydroxyl group.[30-32] When the mutagenicities of sukhteh, or pyrolyzed opium, and of pyrolyzed morphine were compared before and after treatment with nitrous acid, the S9-mediated mutagenicity in both TA98 and TA1538 strains of all three pyrolysates decreased significantly; the mutagenicity of pyrolyzed morphine and opium, as well as sukhteh, was reduced by 46 to 56%, 38 to 42%, and 18%,

Table 5
ESTIMATIONS OF THE CONTRIBUTIONS OF INDIVIDUAL ALKALOIDS TO THE TOTAL S9-MEDIATED
MUTAGENIC ACTIVITY OF PYROLYZED INDIAN OPIUM

Alkaloid	Concentration of alkaloid in crude Indian opium (mg/mg opium)[a]	Amount of condensate (CH_2Cl_2 extract) produced by pyrolysis (mg/mg alkaloid)	Observed mutagenicity (revertants in TA98/mg extract)	Calculated mutagenicity (revertants in TA98/mg opium)	Relative contribution to total mutagenicity (%)
Morphine	0.089	0.29	87,500	2,300	84.1
Thebaine	0.021	0.30	65,500	400	14.6
Codeine	0.126	0.16	1,010	30	1.1
Noscapine	0.126	0.16	230	5	0.2
Papaverine	0.009	0.44	70	0.3	0.01
Total	0.282			2,735.3	
Indian opium		0.23	5,900	1,360	

[a]   Determined by high performance liquid chromatography (HPLC).

From Malaveille, C. et al., *Carcinogenesis*, 3, 577, 1982. With permission.

respectively. The nitrous acid-dependent reduction of the S9-mediated mutagenicity of 2-aminofluorene (control) was 100%. Such data strongly suggest that all three pyrolysates contain primary aromatic amines to a variable extent, which are in part responsible for the mutagenicity of these mixtures.

Several conclusions can be drawn as to the type of compounds involved in the mutagenicity of sukhteh and opium pyrolysates, even though confirmation by spectro-analytical methods is still required.

Conclusion 1. The compounds, after metabolic activation, produce frame-shift mutagens, implying the presence of PAH or heterocyclic derivatives that possess a planar ring-system. This idea is supported by the observation that mutagenicity is as high in TA1538 as in TA98 strain and that nitro and nitroso groups are easily introduced into the molecule through treatment with nitrous acid, yielding nitro-aromatic compounds.[28]

Conclusion 2. Primary aromatic amines and/or heterocyclic (nitrogen-containing) PAH appear to be major mutagenic constituents; mutagenicity increased with the nitrogen content of pyrolyzed opium samples (Figure 2), and deamination by nitrous-acid treatment reduced mutagenicity of the various opium pyrolysates by 18 to 56%. This conclusion is further supported by the observation that the concentration of direct-acting mutagens present in opium pyrolysates is negligible. Both classes of compounds, i.e., aromatic amines and aromatic hydrocarbons, are known to require activation by S9 preparations (through oxidative pathways). Benzo[a]pyrene does not contribute appreciably to the mutagenicity of sukhteh. S9-mediated mutagenicity in TA98 of 1 mg of sukhteh is equivalent to that produced by 3 μg of benzo[a]pyrene (Table 6). However, this compound has been detected in sukhteh at a level 1500 times lower (2 ng benzo[a]pyrene/mg sukhteh).[33]

Conclusion 3. The high mutagenicity of pyrolysates of morphine, thebaine, and codeine (as compared with that of pyrolysates of alkaloids like papaverine, noscapine and narceine) indicates that a tricyclic phenanthrene-type ring system (Figure 3) is required for appreciable mutagenicity to be present after pyrolysis. In addition, the drastic reduction in the mutagenicity of pyrolyzed codeine, as compared with that of morphine (Table 4), indicates that free hydroxyl groups must be present for mutagens to be formed during (mild) pyrolysis.

III. CONCLUSIONS

The bacterial mutagenicities of various pyrolyzed smoke condensates of opium and tobacco, as well as other pyrolyzed naturally-occurring substances to which man may be exposed, are compared in Table 6. The mutagenic activity of sukhteh samples, collected in an area of high esophageal cancer incidence in Iran, was of the same order as that of various tobacco smoke condensates. Opium pyrolyzed in the laboratory had an approximately 10-fold higher mutagenic activity, while the pyrolysates of its major constituent, morphine,

Table 6
RAT LIVER S9-MEDIATED MUTAGENICITY IN
SALMONELLA TYPHIMURIUM **TA98 OF VARIOUS**
PYROLYZED, NATURALLY OCCURRING
SUBSTANCES, COMPARED WITH THAT OF
BENZO[A]PYRENE AND 2-NAPHTHYLAMINE

Material	Range of mutagenicity in *S. typhimurium* strain TA98 (revertants/mg)	Ref.
Sukhteh (CH$_2$Cl$_2$ extract)	70—1540	Table 2
Opium pyrolysate (CH$_2$Cl$_2$ extract)	5900	Table 3
Morphine pyrolysate (CH$_2$Cl$_2$ extract)	87,500	Table 3
Cigarette, cigar, pipe smoke condensate	50—2 000[a]	38 39 40 27 41
Marijuana smoke condensate	500—1600[a]	40 27
D-tryptophan pyrolysate	22,000	42
Joss stick smoke condensate	90—120[a]	43
Benzo[a]pyrene	206,000[b]	28
2-naphthylamine	1800[b]	28

Note: The figures in the table are collated from the literature.

[a] Range of values reported in the literature.
[b] Determined from assays containing 3.4 μg of benzo[a]pyrene or 5 to 40 μg of 2-naphthylamine (concentrations that give linear dose-response curves).

yielded another 10-fold increase in specific mutagenicity. The mutagenic effect of these compounds is relatively high when compared with that of 2-naphthylamine tested under identical conditions, i.e., the pyrolysate of morphine was about 50-fold more mutagenic (see Table 6). By inference, opium pyrolysates must be considered as potentially carcinogenic substances. Investigations to assess the genotoxic potential of these pyrolysates in other short-term tests as well as in long-term carcinogenicity assays in rodents are underway. As already demonstrated, sukhteh and morphine pyrolysates produced in human lymphocytes from peripheral blood a substantial increase of sister chromatid exchanges at concentrations lower than those required for a similar response with cigarette smoke condensate.[34]

In humans, opium smoking has been associated with an increased incidence of cancer of the urinary bladder, particularly in adult men.[35] The findings that primary aromatic amines contribute substantially to the total mutagenicity of sukhteh and of pyrolysates of opium and morphine (of the order of 20 to 50%) may be relevant in this respect; the urinary bladder is the primary target organ for carcinogenic aromatic amines in man.[36]

The main findings of a series of epidemiological and environmental studies in the area in northeast Iran, where there is a high incidence of esophageal cancer, have indicated that the incidence is associated (although causality has not been established) with the use of opium pyrolysates, excessive consumption of hot tea and a restricted diet, in particular, riboflavin deficiency, low intake of vitamins A and C, and of animal protein.

In that high-incidence area, histological abnormalities (esophagitis, atrophic changes of the esophagus) are seen in 80% or more of the population, even from the youngest group studied (i.e., teenagers),[37] indicating widespread insults to the esophagus at a young age. No evidence was found that the food is appreciably contaminated by known carcinogens[12] such as polycyclic hydrocarbons, volatile nitrosamines, or mycotoxins. Nitrate and nitrite levels in food and water were extremely low; tobacco smoking and chewing and consumption of alcohol had an almost negligible role. Even though opium is unlikely to be an important etiological factor in many other parts of the world, the results of this multidisciplinary study indicate an etiology of esophageal cancer which could be of general significance, that is, widespread, frequent direct exposure of the esophagus to genotoxic compounds rendered susceptible by dietary deficiency, possibly in conjunction with other tumor-enhancing stimuli (use of hot tea). This mechanism appears to be analogous to that linking alcohol and cigarette smoking, agents which have been identified as etiological factors in esophageal cancer in other parts of the world.

Both in the Transkei and in northeast Iran, the high incidence is unlikely to result from a single cause. The role of genetic factors, for example, needs further examination, especially in northeast Iran, where, as in the Soviet Union and in Afghanistan, the risk is highest in the Turkic groups. However, although geographic and secular differences in the incidence of the disease may result from the complex interaction of many factors, environmental mutagens/carcinogens are likely to initiate the disease and the mutagenic agents described above are likely candidates in the two areas.

ACKNOWLEDGMENTS

We thank Jean Hawkins and Yvette Granjard for secretarial help. The authors are particularly grateful to the French Ministry of Health and Family for kindly authorizing the purchase and/or importation of many of the materials used in this study. This work was supported in part by contract N01-CP-71048 from the National Cancer Institute, Bethesda, Md., U.S.A.

REFERENCES

1. **Wynder, E. L. and Bross, I. J.,** A study of etiological factors in cancer of the esophagus, *Cancer,* 14, 389, 1961.
2. **Tuyns, A. J., Pequignot, A. J., and Jensen, O. M.,** Le cancer de l'oesophage en Ille-et-Vilaine en fonction des niveaux de consommation d'alcool et de tabac. Des risques qui se multiplient, *Bull. Cancer,* 64, 45, 1977.
3. **Day, N. E. and Muñoz, N.,** Esophagus, in *Cancer Epidemiology and Prevention,* Schottenfeld, D. and Fraumeni, J. F., Eds., W. B. Saunders, Philadelphia, 1982, 596.
4. **Mahboubi, E., Kmet, J., Cook, P. J., Day, N. E., Ghadirian, P., and Salmasizadeh, S.,** Oesophageal cancer studies in the Caspian littoral of Iran: the Caspian cancer registry, *Br. J. Cancer,* 28, 197, 1973.
5. **Nugmanov, S. N. and Kolycheva, N. I.,** Age, sex and ethnic characteristics of patients with esophageal carcinoma in Kazakhstan, in *Epidemiology of Malignant Tumors,* Nauka Press, Alma Ata, 1970, 272.
6. **Rose, E. F. and McGlashan, N. D.,** The spatial distribution of oesophageal cancer in the Transkei, South Africa, *Br. J. Cancer,* 31, 197, 1975.
7. **Tuyns, A. J. and Massé, L. M. F.,** Mortality from cancer of the oesophagus, *Int. J. Cancer,* 2, 241, 1973.
8. **van Rensburg, S. J.,** Epidemiologic and dietary evidence for a specific nutritional predisposition to esophageal cancer, *J. Natl. Cancer Inst.,* 67, 243, 1981.
9. **Rose, E.,** Environmental factors associated with cancer of the oesophagus in Transkei, in *Carcinoma of the Oesophagus,* Silber, W., Ed., Balkema, Rotterdam, 1978, 91.
10. **McGlashan, N. D., Bradshaw, E., and Harington, J. S.,** Cancer of the oesophagus and the use of tobacco and alcoholic beverages in Transkei, 1975-6, *Int. J. Cancer,* 29, 249, 1982.

11. **Hewer, T., Rose, E., Ghadirian, P., Castegnaro, M., Bartsch, H., Malaveille, C., and Day, N. E.,** Ingested mutagens from opium and tobacco pyrolysis products and cancer of the oesophagus, *Lancet,* 2, 494, 1978.

12. Joint Iran/IARC Study Group, Esophageal cancer studies in the Caspian littoral of Iran: results of population studies — a prodrome, *J. Natl. Cancer Inst.,* 54, 1127, 1977.

13. **Cook-Mozaffari, P. J., Azordegan, F., Day, N. E., Ressicaud, A., Sabai, C., and Aramesh, B.,** Oesophageal cancer studies in the Caspian littoral of Iran: results of a case-control study, *Br. J. Cancer,* 39, 293, 1979.

14. **Hormozdiari, H., Day, N. E., Aramesh, B., and Mahboubi, E.,** Dietary factors and esophageal cancer in the Caspian littoral of Iran, *Cancer Res.,* 35, 3493, 1975.

15. **Kmet, J., McLaren, D., and Siassi, F.,** Epidemiology of oesophageal cancer with special reference to nutritional studies among the Turkoman in Iran, in *Advances in Modern Human Nutrition,* Tobin, R. B. and Mehlman, M. A., Eds., Pathotox Publishers, New York, 1980.

16. **Gorodetzky, C.,** Personal communication, 1982.

17. **Wynder, E. L. and Graham, E. A.,** Tobacco smoking as a possible etiologic factor on bronchogenic carcinoma, *JAMA,* 143, 329, 1950.

18. **Doll, R. and Hill, A. B.,** Smoking and carcinoma of the lung, *Br. Med. J.,* 2, 739, 1950.

19. **Wynder, E. L. and Hoffmann, D.,** Tobacco, in *Cancer Epidemiology and Prevention,* Schottenfeld, D. and Fraumeni, J. F., Eds., W. B. Saunders, Philadelphia, 1982, 277.

20. **Stedman, R. L.,** The chemical composition of tobacco and tobacco smoke, *Chem. Rev.,* 68, 153, 1968.

21. **Neurath, G., Pirmann, B., and Wichern, H.,** On the problem of *N*-nitroso compounds in tobacco smoke, *Beitr. Tabakforsch.,* 2, 311, 1964.

22. **Hoffmann, D., Hecht, S. S., Ornaf, R. M., and Wynder, E. L.,** *N*-nitrosonornicotine in tobacco, *Science,* 186, 265, 1974.

23. **Van Duuren, B. L.,** Tobacco carcinogenesis, *Cancer Res.,* 28, 2357, 1968.

24. **Mizusaki, S., Okamoto, H., Akyiama, A., and Fukuhara, Y.,** Relation between chemical constituents of tobacco and mutagenic activity of cigarette smoke condensate, *Mutat. Res.,* 48, 319, 1977.

25. **Matsumoto, I. D., Yoshida, D., Mizusaki, S., and Okamoto, H.,** Mutagenicity on pyrolytic products of amino acids, in *Proceedings of the 5th Annual Meeting of the Environmental Mutagen Society,* Environmental Mutagen Society, Tokyo, 6, 1976.

26. **Sugimura, T., Nagao, N., and Wakabayashi, K.,** Mutagenic heterocyclic amines in cooked food, in *Environmental Carcinogens — Selected Methods of Analysis, Volume 4 — Some Aromatic Amines and Azo Dyes in the General and Industrial Environment,* IARC Sci. Publ. No. 40, Fishbein, L., Castegnaro, M., O'Neill, I. K., and Bartsch, H., Eds., International Agency for Research on Cancer, Lyon, France, 1981, 251.

27. **Wehner, F. C., van Rensburg, S. J., and Thiel, P. G.,** Mutagenicity of marijuana and Transkei tobacco smoke condensates in the *Salmonella*/microsome assay, *Mutat. Res.,* 77, 135, 1980.

28. **Malaveille, C., Friesen, M., Camus, A.-M., Garren, L., Hautefeuille, A., Bereziat, J.-C., Ghadirian, P., Day, N. E., and Bartsch, H.,** Mutagens produced by the pyrolysis of opium and its alkaloids as possible risk factors in cancer of the bladder and esophagus, *Carcinogenesis* 3, 577, 1982.

29. British Pharmaceutical Codex, Opium, 337, 1973.

30. **Tsuda, M., Takahashi, Y., Nagao, M., Hirayama, T., and Sugimura, T.,** Inactivation of mutagens from pyrolysates of tryptophan and glutamic acid by nitrite in acidic solution, *Mutat. Res.,* 78, 331, 1980.

31. **Tsuda, M., Nagao, M., Hirayama, T., and Sugimura, T.,** Nitrite converts 2-amino-α-carboline, an indirect mutagen, into 2-hydroxy-α-carboline, a non-mutagen and 2-hydroxy-3-nitroso-3-carboline, a direct mutagen, *Mutat. Res.,* 83, 61, 1981.

32. **Haugen, D. A., Peak, M. J., and Reilly, C. A.,** Use of nitrous acid-dependent decrease in mutagenicity as an indication of the presence of mutagenic primary aromatic amines - non-specific reactions with phenols and benzo(*a*)pyrene, *Mutat. Res.,* 82, 59, 1981.

33. **Grimmer, G.,** Personal communication, 1981.

34. **Perry, P. E. and Evans, H. J.,** Personal communication, 1982.

35. **Sadeghi, A., Behmard, S., and Vesselinovitch, S. D.,** Opium: a potential urinary bladder carcinogen in man, *Cancer,* 43, 2315, 1979.

36. International Agency for Research on Cancer, *IARC Monographs on the Evaluation of the Carcinogenic Risk of Chemicals to Humans,* Suppl. 1, IARC, Lyon, France, 1979.

37. **Crespi, M., Grassi, A., Amiri, G., Muñoz, N., Aramesh, B., Mojtabai, A., and Casale, V.,** Oesophageal lesions in northern Iran: a premalignant condition? *Lancet,* 2, 217, 1979.

38. **Kier, L. D., Yamasaki, E., and Ames, B. N.,** Detection of mutagenic activity in cigarette smoke condensates, *Proc. Natl. Acad. Sci. U.S.A.,* 71, 4159, 1974.

39. **Sato, S., Seino, Y., Ohka, T., Yahagi, T., Nagao, M., Matsushima, T., and Sugimura, T.,** Mutagenicity of smoke condensates from cigarettes, cigars and pipe tobacco, *Cancer Lett.,* 3, 1, 1977.

40. **Busch, F. W., Seid, D. A., and Wei, E. T.,** Mutagenic activity of marijuana smoke condensates, *Cancer Lett.,* 6, 319, 1979.

41. **Bartsch, H., Malaveille, C., Camus, A.-M., Martel-Planche, G., Brun, G., Hautefeuille, A., Sabadie, N., Barbin, A., Kuroki, T., Drevon, C., Piccoli, C., and Montesano, R.,** Validation and comparative studies on 180 chemicals with *S. typhimurium* strains and V-79 Chinese hamster cells in the presence of various metabolizing systems, *Mutat. Res.,* 76, 1, 1980.

42. **Nagao, M., Honda, M., Seino, Y., Yahagi, T., Kawachi, T., and Sugimura, T.,** Mutagenicities of protein pyrolysates, *Cancer Lett.,* 2, 355, 1977.

43. **Saito, S., Makino, R., Takahashi, Y., Sugimura, T., and Miyazaki, T.,** Mutagenicity of smoke condensates from joss sticks, *Mutat. Res.,* 77, 31, 1980.

Part II
Distribution of Naturally Occurring
Carcinogens and Mutagens

Chapter 7

CARCINOGENS OF PLANT ORIGIN: AN OVERVIEW

Iwao Hirono

TABLE OF CONTENTS

I. INTRODUCTION

Epidemiological data strongly suggest that most human cancers, except occupational cancers, are caused by environmental factors that are closely related to human life and especially food. Carcinogens are known to be present in some plants used as human foods or folk medicines. For instance, cycasin, a toxic glucoside, is present in cycads; bracken contains a carcinogen; and carcinogenic pyrrolizidine alkaloids are present in many species of Compositae, Leguminosae, and other families of plants. These carcinogens are specific compounds that are produced by certain plants. They have been classified as secondary metabolites to distinguish them from primary metabolites which are involved in energy metabolism or assimilation in plants. However, the significance of these carcinogens to the plants in which they are found is still unknown; possibly these secondary metabolites have protective effects as eco-chemicals.

These carcinogens of plant origin are little known, since most carcinogens are found by accident. Many more carcinogenic substances will probably be found in natural sources as studies in this field progress.

II. CARCINOGENS OF PLANT ORIGIN

A. Cycasin and Methylazoxymethanol-β-ᴅ-Glucoside

Studies on the carcinogenic activity of cycasin[1,2] by Laqueur and his co-workers first indicated the importance of intestinal microorganisms in the metabolism of certain carcinogens. Cycasin was isolated from the seeds of *Cycas revoluta* Thunb., identified in 1955 by Nishida et al., and later found by Riggs in *Cycas circinalis* L. from Guam (Figure 1). Since the incidence of amyotrophic lateral sclerosis, a neurological disease, is unusually high on the island of Guam, Laqueur et al. focused attention on the cause of this disease. They found that the cycad, which has long been used as a source of food starch on Guam, when fed to rats as crude cycad meal, induced hepatocellular carcinomas, kidney tumors, and intestinal tumors, but not neurological disorders. Subsequently, they found that the carcinogen in cycads is cycasin. Cycasin is carcinogenic not only to rats but also to other animals as shown in Table 1. Since the acute intoxication induced in humans by cycads showed the symptoms of acute liver damage, as in rats, cycasin also seems to be carcinogenic to humans.

Cycasin was toxic only when given orally, and it was not toxic to germ-free rats. These observations strongly suggested that intestinal microorganisms contain an enzyme that hydrolyzes cycasin in vivo. Germ-free rats were then infected with pure strains of microorganisms with or without β-glucosidase activity. After colonization of the intestine, cycasin was given by stomach tube. Agreement was found between the enzyme activity of the microorganisms and the extent of cycasin hydrolysis. Whereas cycasin was toxic and carcinogenic only after passage through the GI tract, its aglycone methylazoxymethanol (MAM) (Figure 1) was toxic and induced tumors in both conventional and germ-free rats irrespective of its route of administration; MAM was, therefore, the proximate carcinogen. The nonenzymatic methylating activity of MAM was demonstrated early, but more recent studies suggested that in some cases, alcohol dehydrogenase may be involved in its conversion to a methylating agent (Figure 2).[3]

B. Bracken Carcinogen

The carcinogenicity of bracken[2,4,5] was discovered in studies on cattle "bracken-poisoning" and chronic enzootic hematuria. Evans et al.[4,5] found that rats fed a diet containing dry powder of bracken developed multiple ileal adenocarcinomas. Young bracken fern used as a human food in Japan is also strongly carcinogenic in rats and induces not only adenomas

$$O$$
$$\uparrow$$
$$CH_3-N=N-CH_2O-C_6H_{11}O_5$$

Cycasin

$$O$$
$$\uparrow$$
$$CH_3-N=N-CH_2OH$$

Methylazoxymethanol

FIGURE 1. Chemical structure of cycasin and its aglycone, methylazoxymethanol.

and adenocarcinomas of the ileum and cecum, but also sarcomas. In addition to intestinal tumors, it also induces urinary bladder carcinomas. In Japan, bracken fern is usually used as a human food after its astringent taste has been removed by immersing it in boiling water containing wood ash or sodium bicarbonate. Sometimes fresh bracken is pickled in salt and immersed in boiling water before being eaten. The carcinogenic activity of bracken is greatly reduced by both these treatments.

The carcinogen in bracken has still not been identified.[2] Very recently, Pamukcu et al.[6] reported that rats fed a diet containing 0.1% quercetin developed ileal and urinary bladder tumors in as high incidence as rats fed bracken diet and that quercetin may be one of the carcinogens in bracken because it is present in bracken, though in extremely small amounts. However, other workers could not confirm the carcinogenicity of quercetin.[7-9] Flavonoids such as quercetin and kaempferol are widely distributed in plants and are mutagenic in the Ames test and some other short-term tests. Therefore, it is very important that quercetin, shown to be a mutagen in the Ames test, is not carcinogenic.

C. Pyrrolizidine Alkaloids

Interest in pyrrolizidine alkaloids[2,10] was awakened by the death of animals grazing in fields containing plants comprised of toxic pyrrolizidine alkaloids. More than 100 pyrrolizidine alkaloids have been isolated from plants. Of these, about 30 have been proven to be hepatotoxic, mostly in rodents. Pyrrolizidine alkaloids are present in various kinds of plants throughout the world, particularly herbs of the tribe Senecioneae of the family Compositae, tribe Crotalaria of the family Leguminosae, and tribe Heliotropium of the family Boraginaceae. Toxic pyrrolizidine alkaloids are all hepatotoxins and some alkaloids are also toxic to the lung. Some hepatotoxic pyrrolizidine alkaloids induce hepatocellular carcinoma and hemangioendothelial sarcoma of the liver when given orally or i.p. to rats.[2] Although the carcinogenicity of pyrrolizidine alkaloids has long been known, only the very few pure alkaloids shown in Figure 3 have been proven to be carcinogenic. Nevertheless, it is concluded from the results so far obtained that hepatotoxic pyrrolizidine alkaloids are hepatocarcinogenic. For toxicity, the alkaloids must possess the 1-hydroxymethyl-pyrrolizidine

Table 1
CARCINOGENICITY OF CYCASIN[2]

Animal	Tumor sites and histologic types of tumors
Rat[a]	Large intestine (adenoma, adenocarcinoma), kidney (adenoma, nephroblastoma, interstitial tumor, sarcoma); hepatocellular carcinoma was induced by feeding diet containing cycasin
Mouse[a]	Hepatocellular carcinoma
Hamster[a]	Bile duct carcinoma
Guinea pig[b]	Hepatocellular carcinoma, bile duct tumor
Rabbit[b]	Hemangioendothelial sarcoma of the liver
Monkey[b]	Hepatocellular carcinoma, renal carcinoma

[a]   Single oral dose.
[b]   Long-term feeding of diet containing cycasin.

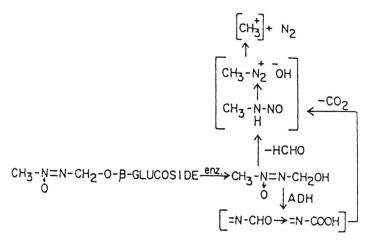

FIGURE 2.   Activation of cycasin under physiological conditions. ADH: alcohol dehydrogenase. (From Miller, E. C. and Miller, J. A., *Accomplishments in Cancer Research 1980,* Fortner, J. G. and Rhoads, J. E., Eds., Lippincott, Philadelphia, 1981. With permission.)

structure, and unsaturation in the 1,2-position, and at least one of the hydroxy groups must be esterified. Pyrrolizidine alkaloids that damage the liver are metabolized in the liver by mixed function oxidase to pyrrolic metabolites that are highly reactive intermediates (Figure 4).

Flowerstalks of *Petasites japonicus* containing petasitenine, *Tussilago farfara* L. containing senkirkine, and *Symphytum officinale* L. (comfrey) containing symphytine are used as human foods and Chinese or folk medicines in Japan.[2] Rats fed a diet containing the dry powder of these plants develop hemangioendothelial sarcoma of the liver, hepatocellular adenoma, and carcinoma. The main malignant hepatic tumors induced by hepatocarcinogenic pyrrolizidine alkaloids are hemangioendothelial sarcomas.

D. Carrageenan

Carrageenan[2] is a sulfated polysaccharide extracted from red seaweeds, including *Chondrus crispus, C. ocellatus, Eucheuma cottonii,* and *E. spinosum*. It is composed of sulfated D-galactose and 3,6-anhydro-D-galactose. The average molecular weight of native carrageenan is 3 to 7 × 10⁵ and it is usually used as a gelling agent, a viscosity builder, or an emulsifying agent. Degraded carrageenan is prepared by acid hydrolysis of native carra-

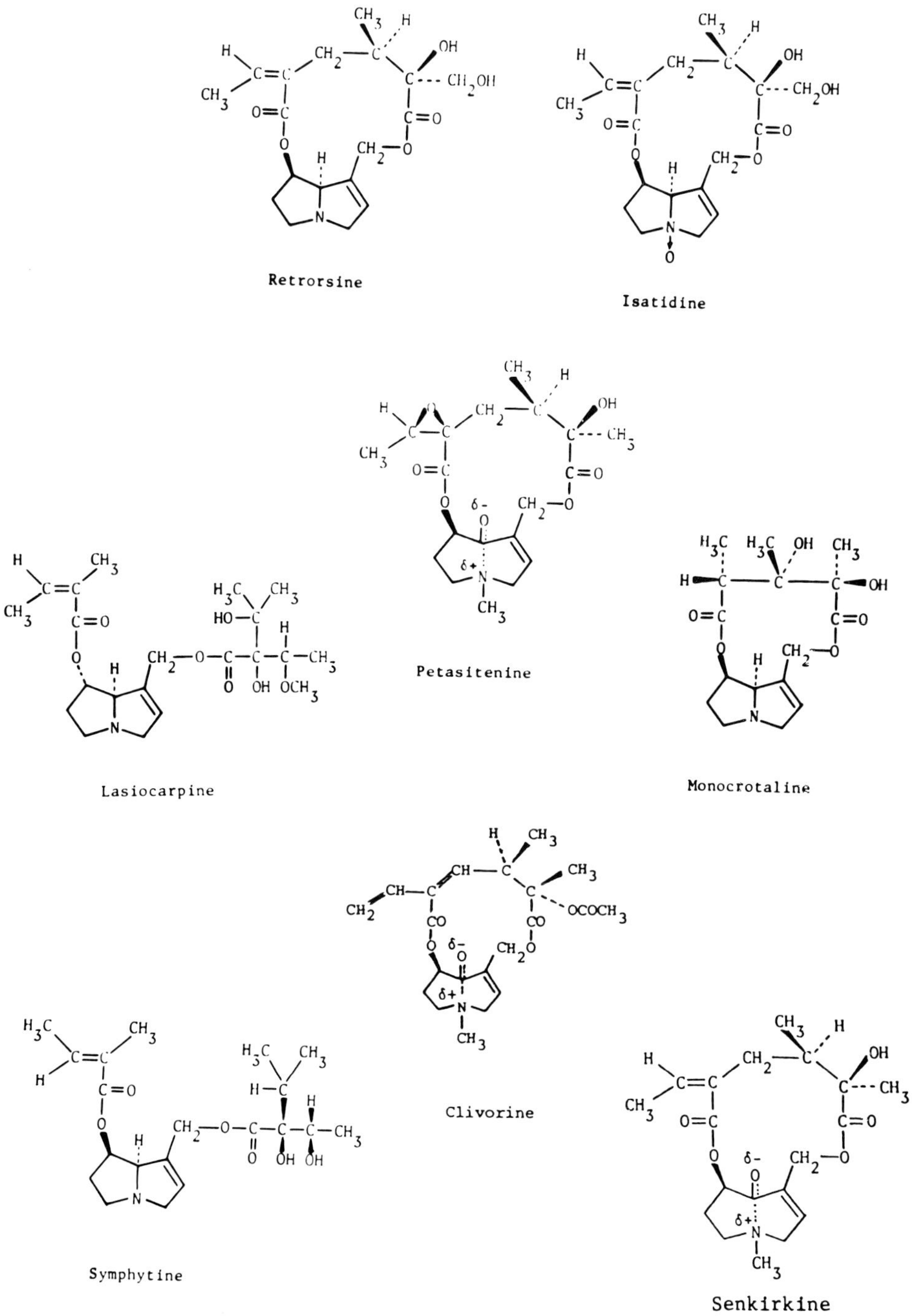

FIGURE 3.   Chemical structure of carcinogenic pyrrolizidine alkaloids.

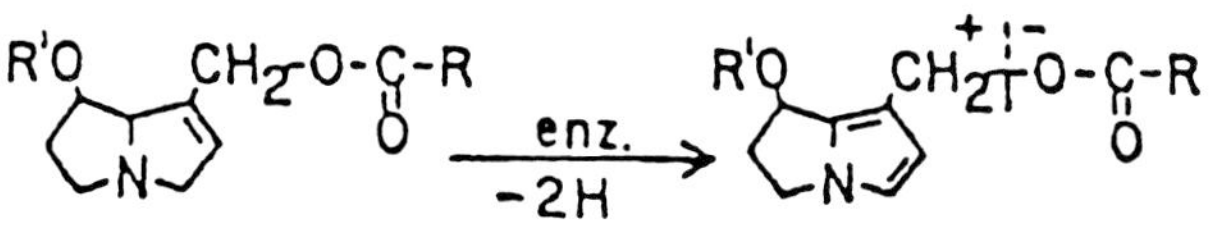

FIGURE 4.   Enzymatic activation of toxic pyrrolizidine alkaloids. (From Miller, E. C. and Miller, J. A., *Accomplishments in Cancer Research 1980,* Fortner, J. G. and Rhoads, J. E., Eds., Lippincott, Philadelphia, 1981. With permission.)

geenan. It has a molecular weight of 2 to 4 $\times$ 10^4 and has been used for therapy of gastric ulcers. Native carrageenan induces sarcomas at the site of s.c. injection in rats, but did not induce tumors when given orally. On the other hand, degraded carrageenan induced adenocarcinomas and squamous cell carcinomas of the large intestine when given orally to rats. The mechanism of the carcinogenic effect of degraded carrageenan is unknown. Since carrageenan is not mutagenic, it is considered to be a nongenotoxic carcinogen. Studies on the carcinogenicity of carrageenan led to those using dextran sulfate sodium which is a readily available well-characterized sulfated polysaccharide, as a nongenotoxic carcinogen.[11] Recently, it was found that mucosal lesions, such as erosion and squamous metaplasia of the large intestine induced by oral administration of degraded carrageenan were more extensive in germ-free rats than in conventional ones. Therefore, bacterial flora are not essential for the biological effects of degraded carrageenan.[12]

E. Other Plant Carcinogens[2]

In addition to the carcinogens described above, it is known that certain carcinogenic hydrazines and their derivatives are present in edible mushrooms, e.g., gyromitrin (acetaldehyde formylmethylhydrazone) in false morel *Gyromitra esculenta* and agaritine (β-*N*-[γ-L(+)-glutamyl]-4-hydroxymethylphenyl-hydrazine) in the cultivated mushroom of Europe and North America *Agaricus bisporus*. Most carcinogens of plant origin described above are present in widely used human foods or herbal remedies. They should not be neglected, even though they are ingested in quite small amounts. Human cancers, other than occupational ones, are thought probably to be due to long-term exposure to small amounts of various kinds of weak carcinogens, rather than to any one potent carcinogen. Thus, the importance of carcinogens of plant origin described here cannot be ignored.

REFERENCES

1. **Laqueur, G. L. and Spatz, M.,** Toxicology of cycasin, *Cancer Res.,* 28, 2262, 1968.
2. **Hirono, I.,** Natural carcinogenic products of plant origin, *CRC Crit. Rev. Toxicol.,* 8, 235, 1981.
3. **Miller, E. C. and Miller, J. A.,** Searches for ultimate chemical carcinogens and their reactions with cellular macromolecules, in *Accomplishments in Cancer Research 1980,* Fortner, J. G. and Rhoads, J. E., Eds., Lippincott, Philadelphia, 1981, 63.
4. **Evans, I. A.,** The radiomimetic nature of bracken toxin, *Cancer Res.,* 28, 2252, 1968.
5. **Evans, I. A.,** The bracken carcinogen, in *Chemical Carcinogens,* Searle, C. E., Ed., ACS Monogr. 173, American Chemical Society, Washington, D.C., 1976, 690.
6. **Pamukcu, A. M., Yalciner, S., Hatcher, J. F., and Bryan, G. T.,** Quercetin, a rat intestinal and bladder carcinogen present in bracken fern *(Pteridium aquilinum), Cancer Res.,* 40, 3468, 1980.
7. **Saito, D., Shirai, A., Matsushima, T., Sugimura, T., and Hirono, I.,** Test of carcinogenicity of quercetin, a widely distributed mutagen in food, *Teratogenesis, Carcinogenesis, Mutagenesis,* 1, 213, 1980.
8. **Hirono, I., Ueno, I., Hosaka, S., Takanashi, H., Matsushima, T., Sugimura, T., and Natori, S.,** Carcinogenicity examination of quercetin and rutin in ACI rats, *Cancer Lett.,* 13, 15, 1981.
9. **Morino, K., Matsukura, N., Kawachi, T., Ohgaki, H., Sugimura, T., and Hirono, I.,** Carcinogenicity test of quercetin and rutin in golden hamsters by oral administration, *Carcinogenesis,* 3, 93, 1982.
10. **Schoental, R.,** Carcinogens in plants and microorganisms, in *Chemical Carcinogens,* ACS Monogr. 173, Searle, C. E., Ed., American Chemical Society, Washington, D.C., 1976, 626.
11. **Hirono, I., Kuhara, K., Hosaka, S., Tomizawa, S., and Golberg, L.,** Induction of intestinal tumors in rats by dextran sulfate sodium, *J. Natl. Cancer Inst.,* 66, 579, 1981.
12. **Hirono, I., Sumi, Y., Kuhara, K., and Miyakawa, M.,** Effect of degraded carrageenan on the intestine in germfree rats, *Toxicol. Lett.,* 8, 207, 1981.

Chapter 8

MUTAGENIC COMPOUNDS CONTAINED IN SEAWEEDS

Howard F. Mower

Seaweeds are not thought to be common constituents of the human diet, but they have been important human food material throughout history for the people of Oceania, those living in countries of Asia bordering the Pacific Ocean, and those in other seacoast areas. Examples of the use of seaweeds in traditional ethnic foods include sushi (cooked rice wrapped in seaweed) eaten in Japan, poki (raw seaweed mixed with uncooked fish, raw onions, peppers, and other vegetables) eaten in Hawaii, kim chee (fermented seaweed and cabbage mixed with chili peppers) eaten in Korea, and seaweed soup eaten in China. Seaweed-derived polysaccharides are also used in modern technology and are components of convenience foods and medicinal preparations of many types. Large numbers of humans could suffer significant exposure to hazardous substances if seaweeds contain significant amounts of mutagenic, genotoxic, or carcinogenic materials.

The red marine algae *(Rhodophyta)* have long been known to contain high concentrations of halogenated compounds.[1] They appear to be a unique source of brominated and iodinated compounds. Ten families representing five orders of red seaweeds (*Nemaliales, Cryptonemiales, Gigartinales, Rhodymeniales* and *Ceramiales*) have been shown to contain a diverse array of halogenated organic compounds.[2] In addition, some seaweeds of the *cyanophyta* and *chlorophyta* also accumulate halogen compounds.[3]

The simplest of the halogen compounds to appear in seaweeds is methyl iodide.[4] This compound is a mutagen, and some evidence exists that it is carcinogenic.[5] It has been detected in *Asparagopsis taxiformis* and similar species and found in elevated amounts in seawater near beds of the brown kelp *Laminaria digitata*.[6]

The essential oil of *Asparagopsis* is composed of 80% bromoform ($CHBr_3$), with carbon tetrabromide (CBr_4) as another major constituent.[7] While the genotoxicity of these brominated compounds is unknown, they, along with methyl iodide, may react with the chloride ion of sea water to produce the corresponding chlorinated compounds, chloroform ($CHCl_3$), carbon tetrachloride (CCl_4) and methyl chloride (CH_3Cl).[8] The first two substances have been reported to be constituents of *Asparagopsis*[2] and are known carcinogens and hepatotoxins.[9] Methyl chloride is the principal halocarbon of the atmosphere, and it has been proposed that marine algae may be a significant source of this material.[8]

The essential oil of *Asparagopsis* species can be as much as 5% of the dry weight of the seaweed.[10] Further investigation of this essential oil has shown that it contains a complex array of polyhalogenated hydrocarbons. Table 1 shows an aggregate of compounds found in *Asparagopsis*, as compiled from several studies.[2,11-13] Seaweed samples were collected from the Gulf of California, from the Caribbean, from Hawaii, and from the Spanish Mediterranean coast *(A. armata)*. Each sample contained most of these substances, but within one region there is some north-south variation in the biosynthesis of these halometabolites, which suggests that environmental influences can alter the halocarbon mixture found in any seaweed sample.

Very few of the substances listed in Table 1 have been tested for mutagenicity. Compounds of the series CCl_3–$COCCl_3$,[14] CCl_3–$COOH$,[15] and CCl_3–CHO are all mutagenic. However, the mutagenicity of the first two compounds results from reactive intermediates formed with dimethyl sulfoxide (DMSO), the solvent usually employed in mutagen testing. Thus their genotoxicity in the absence of this material may be minimal. Polyhaloacetones, bromo- and iodo-acetic acids are effective alkylating agents, combining with and inhibiting enzymes by reaction with sulfhydryl groups of cysteine, the hydroxy groups of serine and threonine,

Table 1
CONSTITUENTS OF *ASPARAGOPSIS* SPECIES

Type of compound	No.	Structure	Estimated % in oil bw
Haloforms	1	$CHBr_3$	80
	2	$CHBr_2I$	5
	3	$CHBrI_2$	2
	4	CHI_3	
	5	$CHBr_2Cl$	
	6	$CHClI_2$	
	7	$CHCl_2$	
	8	$CHCl_3$	
	9	$CHBrCl_2$	
	10	$CHBrClI$	
Dihalomethanes	11	CH_2Br_2	
	12	CH_2BrI	
	13	CH_2I_2	
Carbon tetrahalides	14	CBr_4	
	15	CCl_4	
Carbonyl dihalides	16	COI_2	
2-Haloethanols	17	ICH_2CH_2OH	1
1,2-Dihaloethanes	18	$BrCH_2CH_2I$	
Halogenated acetaldehydes	19	Br_2CHCHO	
Halogenated acetones	20	CH_3COCH_2Br	
	21	CH_3COCH_2I	
	22	$CH_3COCHBr_2$	2
	23	$BrCH_2COCH_2Br$	
	24	$BrCH_2COCH_2I$	
	25	CH_3COCBr_3	1
	26	CH_3COCBr_2Cl	
	27	$BrCH_2COCHBr_2$	
	28	$ICH_2COCHBr_2$	
	29	$Br_2CHCOCHBr_2$	
	30	$Cl_3CCOCCl_3$	
	31	$ClBrCHCOCH_2Br$	
	32	$ClBrCHCOCHBr_2$	
	33	$BrCH_2COCH_2Cl$	
	34	$ClCH_2COCH_2I$	
	35	$ClBrCHCOCHClBr$	
	36	$Cl_2CHOCHBr_2$	
	37	$Cl_2CHOCHClBr$	
	38	$ClBrCHCOCH_2Cl$	
	39	Cl_2CHOCH_2Br	
	40	$Cl_2CHCOCHCl_2$	
	41	$ClCH_2COCH_2Cl$	
	42	$ClCH_2COCHCl_2$	
	43	$ClCH_2COCHBr_2$	
Halogenated 2-acetoxypropanes	44	$BrCH_2CH(OAc)CHBr_2$	
	45	$Br_2CHCH(OAc)CHBr_2$	
Dihaloisopropanols	46	$Br_2CHCH(OH)CH_3$	
	47	$BrCH_2CH(OH)CH_2Br$	
	48	$ClCH_2CH(OH)CH_2I$	
	49	$BrCH_2CH(OH)CH_2I$	0.01
	50	$ICH_2CH(OH)CH_2I$	0.009
Trihaloisopropanols	51	$BrClCHCH(OH)CH_2Cl$	
	52	$Cl_2CHCH(OH)CH_2Br$	
	53	$BrClCHCH(OH)CH_2Br$	0.01
	54	$Br_2CHCH(OH)CH_2Cl$	0.09
	55	$Br_2CHCH(OH)CH_2Br$	0.3
	56	$BrClCHCH(OH)CH_2I$	0.03
	57	$Br_2CHCH(OH)CH_2I$	0.03

Table 1 (continued)
CONSTITUENTS OF *ASPARAGOPSIS* SPECIES

Type of compound	No.	Structure	Estimated % in oil bw
Tetrahaloisopropanols	58	$Cl_2CHCH(OH)CHCl_2$	
	59	$BrClCHCH(OH)CHCl_2$	
	60	$Br_2CHCH(OH)CHCl_2$	
	61	$Br_2CHCH(OH)CHBrCl$	
	62	$Br_3CCH(OH)CH_2Cl$	
	63	$Br_2CHCH(OH)CHBr_2$	0.30
	64	$Br_2CHCH(OH)CHBrI$	0.03
	65	$Br_2CHCH(OH)CHI_2$	0.007
Halogenated 1,2-epoxypropanes	65	$BrCH_2CHCHBr_2$	
1,1,3,3-Tetrahalopropenes	66	$Br_2C = CHCHBr_2$	2
	67	$Br_2C = CHCHBrCl$	
	68	$Br_2C = CHCHCl_2$	
	69	$BrIC = CHCHBr_2$	
3,3-Dihaloacroleins	70	$Br_2C = CHCHO$	
Halogenated butenones	71	$Br_2C = CHCOCH_3$	
	72	$Br_2C = CHCOCH_2Br$	
	73	$Br_2C = CHCOCH_2I$	
	74	$Br_2C = CHCOCHBr_2$	2
	75	$Br_2C = CHCOCHBrCl$	
	76	$BrClC = CHCOCHBr_2$	
	77	$Cl_2C = CHCOCHBr_2$	
	78	$BrClC = CHCOCHBrCl$	
1,4,4-Trihalobut-3-en-2-ols[c]	79	$Br_2C = CHCH(OH)CH_2Cl$	0.01
	80	$Br_2C = CHCH(OH)CH_2Br$	0.03
1,1,4,4-Tetrahalobut-3-en-2-ols[c]	81	$Br_2C = CHCH(OH)CHCl_2$	
	82	$Cl_2C = CHCH(OH)CHBr_2$	
	83	$Br_2C = CHCH(OH)CHBrCl$	
	84	$BrClC = CHCH(OH)CHBr_2$[d]	0.03
	85	$Br_2C = CHCH(OH)CHBr_2$	0.6
1,1,1,4,4-Pentahalobut-3-en-2-ols[c]	86	$Br_2C = CHCH(OH)CBr_3$	0.04
Dihaloacetamides	87	$BrClCHONH_2$	0.2
	88	$Br_2CHCONH_2$	0.7
	89	$ClICHCONH_2$	0.06
	90	$BrICHCONH_2$	0.5
	91	$I_2CHCONH_2$	0.3
Haloacetic acids	92	$ClCH_2CO_2H$	
	93	$BrCH_2CO_2H$	
	94	ICH_2CO_2H	
Dihaloacetic acids	95	Cl_2CHCO_2H	
	96	$BrClCHCO_2H$	
	97	$ClICHCO_2H$	
	98	Br_2CHCO_2H	
	99	$BrICHCO_2H$	
	100	I_2CHCO_2H	
Trihaloacetic acid	101	Br_3CCOOH	
Haloacrylic acids	102	$ClCH = CHCO_2H$ or $CH_2 = CClCO_2H$	
	103	$BrCH = CHCO_2H$	
	104	$ICH = CHCO_2H$ or $CH_2 = ClCO_2H$	
Dihaloacrylic acids	105	$Cl_2C = CHCO_2H$ or $CHCl = CClCO_2H$	
	106	$BrCH = CHBrCO_2OH$	

Table 1 (continued)
CONSTITUENTS OF *ASPARAGOPSIS* SPECIES

Type of compound	No.	Structure	Estimated % in oil bw
	107	$Br_2CH=CHCO_2H$	
	108	$BrIC=CHCO_2H$	
		$CHBr=CICO_2H$	
		or $CHI=CBrCO_2H$	
	109	$I_2C=CHCO_2H$	
		or $CHI=CICO_2H$	
Trihaloacrylic acids	110	$Br_2C=CBrCO_2H$	
	111	$BrIC=CBrCO_2H$	
		or $Br_2C=CICO_2H$	

Table 2
MUTAGENICITY OF SOME POLYHALOGENATED OCTADIENES OBTAINED FROM MARINE ALGAE

Compound	Maximum colonies/plate [TA100-(S9)]	Concentration µg/plate
$BrCH_2-CCl-CH=CH-CHCl-CClCH=CHBr$ $\quad\;\; CH_3 \qquad\qquad CH_3$	270	50
$BrCH_2-CCl-CH=CH-CHCl-CClCH=CHCl$ $\quad\;\; CH_3 \qquad\qquad CH_3$	253	50
$BrCH_2-CCl-CH=CH-CHCl-CCl-CH=CHCl$ $\quad\;\; CH_2Cl \qquad\qquad CH_3$	154	20
$BrCH_2-CCl-CH=CH-CHCl-CCl-CH=CHBr$ $\quad\;\; CH_2Cl \qquad\qquad CH_3$	135	10
$ClCH_2-CHBr-CCl-CH=CCl-C-C=CH_2$ $\qquad\qquad CH_3 \qquad\quad O\;\; CH_3$	370	20

and the amino groups of lysine and histidine.[16] Compounds with this type of chemical reactivity can be expected to combine with nucleophilic centers of DNA and cause mutations. It is not surprising that extracts of *Asparagopsis* are usually mutagenic, causing reversion of *Salmonella typhimurium* strain TA100 in the absence of rat liver microsomes.[17] Furthermore, considering the genotoxicity and carcinogenicity of vinyl chloride $CH_2=CHCl$, vinylidene chloride $CH_2=CCl_2$, chloroprene $CH_2=CH-CCl=CH_2$, dibromochloropropane $CH_2Br-CHBr-CH_2Cl$, ethylene dibromide $CHBr=CHBr$, acrolene $CH_2=CH-CHO$, and acetamide CH_3CONH_2, etc., it is quite easy to believe that many of the substances in Table 1 would be hazardous to human health.

In Hawaii, *Asparagopsis taxiformis* is called limu kohu, which means "the supreme seaweed". Japanese in Hawaii refer to it as ogo. It is highly prized for its aroma and flavor.[18] Beaches where the seaweed is abundant are often crowded with persons harvesting the algae. Whether consumption of this seaweed contributes to the cancer incidence in Hawaii is a question that will have to be further studied. It should be pointed out, however, that Hawaiians have one of the highest cancer incidences of any minority group living in the U.S., and the incidence of liver cancer in this group is higher than the U.S. average.

Another red marine algae, *Plocamium*, has been studied for the natural products it contains.[19] Five acyclic halogenated products were isolated and are shown in Table 2. These compounds were tested for mutagenicity, and all five induced revertants in *Salmonella typhimurium* strains TA100 and TA1535 in the absence of rat liver microsomes. The cross-conjugated ketone was the most mutagenic compound of the group and was approximately 200 times more active (revertants per nanomole) at 15 μg per plate as ethyl methanesulfonate, which was used as a positive control in this study.

Progress in this field has been greatly aided by the development of gas chromatography and the interface of GC columns to mass spectrometers. Table 1 is eloquent testimony to the power of this technique, especially when one considers that some of these compounds are present in trace amounts. To measure the mutagenicity of these substances requires several orders of magnitude more material than for their structure assignment by gas chromatography/mass spectrometry. The complete understanding of the genotoxicity of the components of the red algae must await the development of micromutation assay systems. However, many interesting mutagenic substances are certainly to be discovered in seaweeds.

REFERENCES

1. **Fencial, W.,** Halogenation in the *Rhodophyta* - a review, *J. Phycol.,* 11, 245, 1975.
2. **McConnell, O. and Fencial, W.,** Halogen chemistry of the red alga *Asparagopsis, Phytochemistry,* 16, 367, 1977.
3. **Pedersen, M. and Da Silva, E. J.,** Simple brominated phenols in the bluegreen alga *Calothrix brevissima* West, *Planta,* 115, 83, 1973.
4. **Lovelock, J. E.,** Natural halocarbons in the air and in the sea, *Nature (London),* 256, 193, 1975.
5. **McCann, J., Choi, E., Yamasaki, E., and Ames, B. N.,** Detection of carcinogens as mutagens in the *Salmonella*/microsome test: assay of 300 chemicals, *Proc. Natl. Acad. Sci. U.S.A.,* 72, 5135, 1975.
6. **Lovelock, J. E., Maggs, R. J., and Wade, R. J.,** Halogenated hydrocarbons in and over the Atlantic, *Nature (London),* 241, 195, 1974.
7. **Burreson, B. J., Moore, R. E., and Roller, P.,** Haloforms in the essential oil of the alga *Asparagopsis taxiformis (Rhodophyta), Tetrahedron Lett.,* 7, 473, 1975.
8. **Zafiriou, O. C.,** Reaction of methyl halides with sea water and marine aerosols, *J. Mar. Res.,* 33, 75, 1975.
9. **Reuber, M. D. and Glover, E. L.,** Cirrhosis and carcinomas of the liver in male rats given subcutaneous carbon tetrachloride, *J. Natl. Cancer Inst.,* 44, 419, 1970.
10. **Fencial, W.,** Natural products chemistry in the marine environment, *Science,* 215, 923, 1982.
11. **Burreson, B. J., Moore, R. E., and Roller, P. P.,** Volatile halogen compounds in the alga *Asparagopsis taxiformis (Rhodophyta), J. Agric. Food Chem.,* 24, 856, 1976.
12. **Woolard, F. X., Moore, R. E., and Roller, P. P.,** Halogenated acetic and acrylic acids from the red alga *Asparagopsis taxiformis, Phytochemistry,* 15, 617, 1979.
13. **Woolard, F. X. and Moore, R. E.,** Halogenated acetamides, but-3-en-2ols and isopropanols from *Asparagopsis taxiformis* (Delile) Trev., *Tetrahedron,* 32, 2846, 1976.
14. **Zochlinski, H. and Mower, H.,** The mutagenic properties of hexachloroacetone in short-term bacterial mutagen assay systems, *Mutat. Res.,* 89, 137, 1981.
15. **Nestmann, E. R., Chu, I., Kowbel, D. J., and Matula, T. I.,** Short-lived mutagen in *Salmonella* produced by reaction of trichloroacetic acid in dimethylsulphoxide, *Can. J. Genet. Cytol.,* 22, 35, 1980.
16. **Friedman, R. B.,** Applications of the chemical reactions of proteins in studies of their structure and function, *Q. Rev.,* 25, 431, 1961.
17. **Mower, H. F. and Moore, R. E.,** unpublished data.
18. **Abbott, A. and Williamson, E. H.,** *Limu (An Ethnobotanical Study of Some Edible Hawaiian Seaweeds),* Pacific Tropical Botanical Garden, Lawai, Kauai, Hawaii, 1974.
19. **Leary, J. V., Kfir, R., Sims, J. J., and Fulbright, D. W.,** The mutagenicity of natural products from marine algae, *Mutat. Res.,* 68, 301, 1979.

Chapter 9

PHOTOSENSITIZING PLANT PRODUCTS

Gerald A. Poulton and Michael J. Ashwood-Smith

TABLE OF CONTENTS

I. INTRODUCTION

Naturally occurring plant products which result in sensitization in other living systems have received a great deal of attention recently. Several recent reviews have summarized the photodynamic action and photosensitizing abilities of many such compounds; an extensive review by Towers[1] covers the literature prior to 1980, dealing not only with those plant materials having direct photosensitizing properties, but also those which exhibit indirect activity. More specific reviews on contact dermatitis[2-4] have also appeared. This interest in photosensitizing properties has also led naturally to the development of new laboratory methods for the evaluation and quantitative comparison of the effect of various compounds. Kaidbey and Kligman[5,6] have described human tests for the evaluation of topically applied agents as did Weinberg and Springer[7] (on fragrance materials) while Schimmer et al. described photomutagenicity and phototoxicity tests with *Chlamydomonas reinhardii*.[8]

This review will concentrate on the literature since 1980 that has not been extensively reviewed, and will present the data in tabular form, organized by a structural classification.

II. HETEROCYCLIC OXYGEN COMPOUNDS

By far the most extensively studied of the photosensitizing plant products, coumarins and furocoumarins have been the subject of many excellent reviews[9-12] and at least one international conference.[13] These compounds are known to intercalate with DNA to form stable complexes,[14-17] to undergo photocycloaddition with nucleic acids,[18,19] and to produce singlet oxygen under photoexcitation.[20,21] Interest in the photosensitizing properties of these classes of compounds stems from their use in psoralen-UVA (PUVA) therapy for psoriasis and related skin disorders and from their use in suntan preparations resulting from stimulation of melanin production (see for example Song et al.[9] or Magnus and Young[22]).

A. Coumarins

Coumarin and coumarin derivatives have been explored recently for their use as photosensitizing agents in cosmetics, sunscreens, and perfumes.[23] Limettin (5,7-dimethoxycoumarin, 3), naturally occurring in oil of bergamot, shows typical photoproperties, forming excited singlet and triplet states, intercalating with DNA, producing cyclobutane photoadducts with thymidine, but showing much lower toxic potential due to the lack of cross-linking (see below).[23,24] Recent results are summarized in Table 1.

B. Furocoumarins: Psoralens and Angelicins

Furocoumarins have long been used in treatment of psoriasis, vitiligo, and other related skin diseases, and have been shown to produce increased pigmentation in human and guinea pig skin.[9] Recently, however, evidence has mounted that these same compounds cause cell mutation and death, along with a variety of other genetic damage, as a result of UV illumination.[9-12] This photosensitization is known to result both from free furocoumarin (which can generate singlet oxygen by energy transfer from the triplet excited state[20,21]) and from DNA-complexed furocoumarins which can form monoadducts and DNA cross-links,[28,29] although the mechanisms responsible for the observed damage are as yet not completely defined. Angelicin derivatives (furo[3.2,h]coumarins), unlike psoralens (furo[3.2,g]-coumarins), cannot form photocrosslinks in DNA, and thus have been shown not to cause photosensitization after single exposures.[30] Kinetic[31] and theoretical[17] studies, studies on the photocycloaddition reaction[18,19] and the properties of the photoproducts,[32] and comparisons of the photobiological properties of linear and angular furocoumarins[30,33,34] are among the approaches taken to further elucidate the mechanism of furocoumarin photosensitization. Rodighiero[35] has attempted to utilize these data in identifying monofunctional agents which may serve usefully in therapy. Recent literature data, including those showing the effects of furocoumarins on lens proteins[36] and tryptophan metabolism[37,38] are summarized in Table 2.

Table 1
BIOLOGICAL EFFECTS INDUCED BY
COUMARINS AND LIGHT

Test/system	Compound	Ref.
Model studies	13	18,26
Mutation induction, hamster, *Escherichia coli*	3	24
Mutation induction, *Saccharomyces cerevisiae*	3	27
Photosensitization, allergy in man	1,2,3	23
Phototoxicity, hamster, *Escherichia coli*	3	24

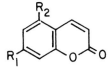

1 $R_1=R_2=H$
2 $R_1=OMe, R_2=H$
3 $R_1=R_2=OMe$

C. Pyranocoumarins, Chromones

Pyranocoumarins (e.g., xanthoxyletin, 16, and xanthyletin, 17) having approximately the same molecular configuration as the psoralens, can intercalate with DNA and undergo photoaddition reactions leading to similar photosensitizing properties (see Table 2). Furo-chromones (e.g., visnagin, 14, and khellin, 15), on the other hand, may intercalate with DNA effectively but cannot form suitable cross-links and are thus less photosensitizing.

III. POLYACETYLENES AND POLYACETYLENE-DERIVED COMPOUNDS

Unlike furocoumarins, polyacetylene compounds do not form DNA complexes or cross-links,[66,67] nor do they result in chromosomal damage;[68] their high phototoxicity and biocidal activity have been shown to result from photoactivation (< 400 nm) of noncomplexed molecules[69] producing free radicals[67] whose target is most likely the cell membranes.[66] The mode of action of α-terthienyl (18), a polyacetylene photosensitizer, is much less well defined. Towers[70] and Gommers et al.[71,72] have shown that α-terthienyl's photosensitivity is enhanced by oxygen, that it is rendered less toxic by singlet oxygen scavengers, and that the harmful effects are related to the inactivation of enzymes by singlet oxygen-derived pathways; Kagan and co-workers,[73,74] on the other hand, have equated the action of α-terthienyl to that of the psoralens, showing DNA complexation and enhanced toxicity in anaerobic conditions. Clearly more work is required before the complete story is known. Photobiological effects of polyacetylenes are summarized in Table 3; the literature prior to 1980 has been previously reviewed.[1]

IV. HETEROCYCLIC NITROGEN COMPOUNDS

A. Quinolines, Furoquinolines

Many species of the *Rutaceae* are known to cause photodermatitis in man and phototoxicity toward many microorganisms, this activity being attributed to the presence therein of a variety of linear furocoumarins (psoralens). Recently, however, alkaloidal constituents have been also shown to have phototoxic effects similar to, although qualitatively smaller than,

Table 2
BIOLOGICAL EFFECTS INDUCED BY FURO- AND PYRANO-COUMARINS AND FUROCHROMONES AND LIGHT

Test/system	Compound	Ref.
Phototoxicity, growth inhibition, mutagenicity		
Bacillus subtilis	5,6	39
Candida albicans	5,6,11	40
Candida utilis	5	41
Chlamydomonas reinhardii	5,6,8—11,14,16	8,42
Escherichia coli	4,5,6,11	29,33,34,43—48
Hamster	4,5,6,11	34,43,44,47,49—52
Man	4,5,6,11	34,50,53,54
Mouse	6	22
Paramecium caudatum	5,6	40
Penicillium expansum	4—8,11—15	56
Saccharomyces cerevisiae	4,5	7,27,45,57
Salmonella typhimurium	11	25
Tetrahymena pyriformis	5,6	40
T4BO[r1]	5	58
Dermatitic activity		
Man	6	3,60
Wistar albino rat	4	38
mRNA template activity		
TMV	5	61
Photobinding		
BSA	4,5,11,15	14,62
DNA	4—6,11—15,17	14,15,16,28,30,35,63,64,65
Theoretical studies	4,5	17,28,31
Photoadduct formation		
Man	5	36
Model studies	4,5,6	16,19,64,65
Singlet oxygen generation		
Escherichia coli	5	20
Model studies	4—7,11	21
Tryptophan metabolism		
Guinea pig	4	37
Wistar albino rat	4	38
Colony forming ability		
Trichophyton mentagrophytes	5	59

4 $R_1 = R_2 = H$
5 $R_1 = H$, $R_2 = OMe$
6 $R_1 = OMe$, $R_2 = H$
7 $R_1 = R_2 = OMe$
8 $R_1 = H$, $R_2 = OCH_2CH=C(CH_3)_2$
9 $R_1 = H$, $R_2 = OH$

11 $R_1 = R_2 = H$
12 $R_1 = R_2 = OMe$
13 $R_1 = H$, $R_2 = OMe$

10

14 $R_1 = OMe$, $R_2 = H$
15 $R_1 = R_2 = OMe$

16 $R_1 = OCH_3$
17 $R_1 = H$

Table 3
BIOLOGICAL EFFECTS INDUCED BY POLYACETYLENE DERIVATIVES AND LIGHT

Test/system	Compound	Ref.
Photoxicity, growth inhibition, mutagenicity		
Aedes aegypti	18—22,24—27,29—46	69,75
Aphelenchus avenae	18	71
Caenorhabditis elegans	18—20,22,24—26,29—32,34,35,37	75
Candida utilis	18,28	41,73,74
Escherichia coli	18,24,28	67,70,73,74
Man	18,23,24,26,36,45	66
MCMV	24	58
PM2	24	58
Saccharomyces cerevisiae	18,24,28	67,70,73
Simulium vittatum	18—20,22,24—26,29—32,34,35,37	75
Syrian hamster	18,24,38,41,44,45	68
T4BO[r1]	24	58
Singlet oxygen generation		
Glucose-6-P dehydrogenase deactivation	18	72
Photobinding		
DNA	18	74

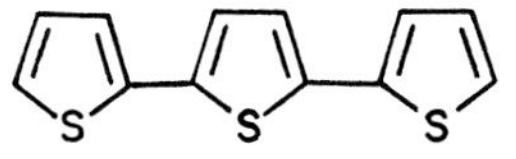

18

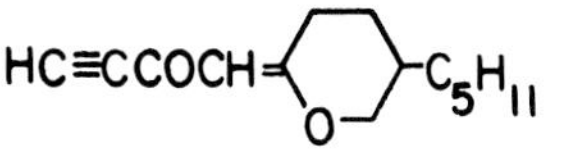

19

$Ph–(C{\equiv}C)–_nR$

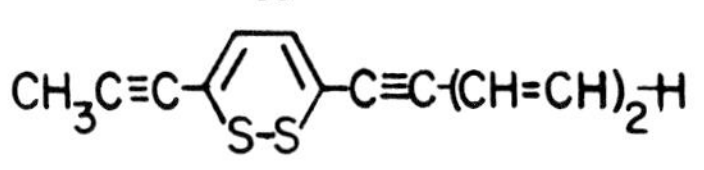

20

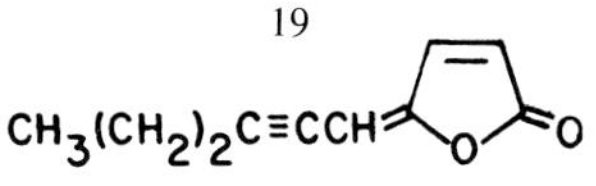

21

$CH_2=CH–(CH_2)_5–CH=CHCH_2–(C{\equiv}C)_2–COCH=CH_2$
22

$CH_2=CHCH(OH)–(C{\equiv}C)_2–CH(OH)CH=CH–(CH_2)_6–CH_3$
23

24:n = 3 R = $–CH_3$
25:n = 2 R = $–CH=CHCHO$
26:n = 2 R = $CH=CH–CH_2OH$
27:n = 3 R = $–CH_2OH$
28:n = 2 R = $–Ph$

$CH_3–(C{\equiv}C)–_n(CH=CH)–_mR$

29: n = 3 m = 2 R = $–(CH_2)_3OCOCH=CMe_2$
30: n = 3 m = 2 R = $–CH(OH)CH_2CH_2OH$

31 n = 3 m = 1 R =

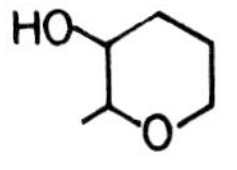

32 n = 3 m = 1 R =

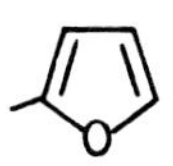

33 n = 2 m = 0 R =

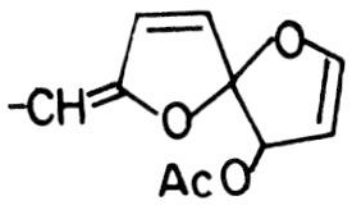

34        $CH_3–(CH=CH)_\ell–(C{\equiv}C)–_m(CH=CH)–_nR$

Table 3 (continued)
BIOLOGICAL EFFECTS INDUCED BY POLYACETYLENE DERIVATIVES AND LIGHT

Test/system	Compound	Ref.
35 $\ell=1$ m$=1$ n$=0$ R$=$		
36 $\ell=1$ m$=1$ n$=0$ R$=$		

37: $\ell=1$ m$=2$ n$=2$ R$=-CH_2CH_2CH_2OAc$
38: $\ell=1$ m$=2$ n$=3$ R$=H$
39: $\ell=1$ m$=2$ n$=2$ R$=-CH(OH)CH_2CH_2OH$
40: $\ell=1$ m$=2$ n$=1$ R$=-CH(OH)CH(OH)CH=CH_2$
41: $\ell=2$ m$=1$ n$=2$ R$=-(CH_2)_5OAc$
42: $\ell=1$ m$=3$ n$=1$ R$=-CH(Cl)CH_2OH$
43: $\ell=1$ m$=2$ n$=2$ R$=-(CH_2)_4CH=CH_2$
44: $\ell=1$ m$=2$ n$=0$ R$=-CH_2CH=CH-(CH_2)_5CH=CH_2$
45: $\ell=1$ m$=3$ n$=1$ R$=-CH(OH)CH_2OH$
46: $\ell=1$ m$=2$ n$=2$ R$=CH(OAc)CH_2CH_2OAc$

the psoralens[76,77] (see Table 4). The suggestion was made[45] that the furoquinoline alkaloids, being similar in size and shape to the psoralens, would have a similar mode of action, a suggestion confirmed by recent work of Ashwood-Smith and co-workers.[78] These compounds therefore form DNA monoadducts,[78] induce sister-chromatid exchanges,[78] but do not appear to attack membrane targets.[76]

B. Other Heterocyclic Compounds

Photodynamic dyes that have been utilized since the 1930s for the inactivation of viruses, particularly the herpes simplex virus, are generally positively-charged and hydrophilic in nature.[83] Snipes[79,80,83] has recently investigated the use of neutral hydrophobic photosensitizing dyes, particularly acridine (60), and has shown that they sensitize lipid containing viruses to near UV radiation in the presence of oxygen. Both DNA damage (irreparable)[80] and membrane damage (which may be repaired)[79] are involved.

Pterins (e.g., 61) are widely distributed throughout the plant and animal kingdom, and are suspected of involvement in a variety of photobiological and phytophysical processes. A recent report[81] has shown that pterins are photosensitizing agents, utilizing either the excited triplet state directly, the production of singlet oxygen, or both.

Table 4
BIOLOGICAL EFFECTS INDUCED BY VARIOUS
HETEROCYCLICS AND LIGHT

Test/system	Compound	Ref.
Toxicity, mutagenicity, growth inhibition		
Bacillus subtilis	47—60	45
Candida albicans	47—60	45
Escherichia coli	47—60	45,78—80
Hamster	47	78
Proteus mirabilis	47—60	45
Pseudomonas fluorescens	47—60	45
Saccharomyces cerevisiae	47—60	45
Staphylococcus albus	47—60	45
Streptococcus faecalis	47—60	45
Singlet oxygen generation		
Model studies	61	81,82
Viral inactivation		
Herpes simplex, φ2, PM2	60	83
Photobinding, photocrosslinking		
DNA	47	76—78

47 R_1 = OMe, R_2 = R_3 = R_4 = H
48 R_1 = R_3 = R_4 = OMe, R_2 = H
49 R_1 = R_4 — OMc, R_3 = OH, R_2 = H
50 R_1 = R_2 = R_3 = OMe, R_4 = H
51 R_1 = R_2 = R_4 = OMe, R_3 = H
52 R_1 = OMe, R_2,R_3 = —OCH$_2$O—, R_4 = H
53 R_1 = R_4 = OMe, R_2,R_3 = —OCH$_2$O—

54 R_1 = —C(OH)—CH$_2$OAc, with CH$_3$

55 R_1 = —C(OH)—CH$_2$OH; HCl salt, with CH$_3$

56

57

58

59

60

61

REFERENCES

1. **Towers, G. H. N.,** Photosensitizers from plants and their photodynamic action, *Prog. Phytochem.,* 6, 183, 1980.
2. **Evans, F. J. and Schmidt, R. J.,** Plants and plant products that induce contact dermatitis, *Planta Med.,* 38, 289, 1980.
3. **Bleehen, S. S.,** Light, chemicals, and the skin: contact photodermatitis, *Br. J. Dermatol.,* 105(Suppl. 21), 23, 1981.
4. **Baer, R. L. and Bickers, D. R.,** Allergic contact dermatitis, photoallergic contact dermatitis, and phototoxic dermatitis, *Comp. Immunol.,* 7, 259, 1981.
5. **Kaidbey, K. H. and Kligman, A. M.,** Identification of topical photosensitizing agents in humans, *J. Invest. Dermatol.,* 70, 149, 1978.
6. **Kaidbey, K. H. and Kligman, A. M.,** Identification of systemic phototoxic drugs by human intradermal assay, *J. Invest. Dermatol.,* 70, 272, 1978.
7. **Weinberg, E. H. and Springer, S. T.,** The evaluation *in vitro* of fragrance materials for phototoxic activity, *J. Soc. Cosmet. Chem.,* 32, 303, 1981.
8. **Schimmer, O., Beck, R., and Dietz, U.,** Phototoxicity and photomutagenicity of furocoumarins and medical plants with furocoumarins in *Chlamydomonas reinhardii.* Comparison of biological activities as a basis of risk evaluation, *Planta Med.,* 40, 68, 1980.
9. **Song, P.-S. and Tapley, K. J.,** Photochemistry and photobiology of psoralens, *Photochem. Photobiol.,* 29, 1177, 1979.
10. **Parsons, B. J.,** Psoralen photochemistry, *Photochem. Photobiol.,* 32, 813, 1980.
11. **Grekin, D. A. and Epstein, J. H.,** Psoralens, UVA (PUVA) and photocarcinogenesis, *Photochem. Photobiol.,* 33, 957, 1981.
12. **Hearst, J. E.,** Psoralen photochemistry, *Annu. Rev. Biophys. Bioeng.,* 10, 69, 1981.
13. **Cahn, J., Forlot, P., Grupper, C., Meybeck, A., and Urbach, F., Eds.,** *Psoralens in Cosmetics and Dermatology,* Pergamon Press, Elmsford, N.Y., 1981.
14. **Beaumont, P. C., Land, E. J., Navaratnam, S., Parsons, B. J., and Phillips, G. O.,** A pulse radiolysis study of the complexing of furocoumarins with DNA and proteins, *Biochem. Biophys. Acta,* 608, 182, 1980.
15. **Sherman, W. V. and Grossweiner, L. I.,** Photobinding of psoralen and 8-methoxypsoralen to calf thymus DNA, *Photochem. Photobiol.,* 34, 579, 1981.
16. **Arnaud, R., Deflandre, A., Lang, G., and Lemaire, J.,** Propriétés photosensibilisatrices des furocoumarines. Étude des furocoumarines angulaires, *C. R. Acad. Sci. Ser. C,* 290, 263, 1980.
17. **Huang, H. H.,** Chemical reaction of DNA with cross-linking agents: influences of base permutation on chemical reactivity, *J. Theoret. Biol.,* 87, 585, 1980.
18. **Shim, S. C., Koh, H. Y., and Chi, D. Y.,** Photocycloaddition reaction of 5,7-dimethoxycoumarin to thymidine, *Photochem. Photobiol.,* 34, 177, 1981.
19. **Hahn, B. S., Joshi, P. C., Kan, L. S., and Wang, S. Y.,** Heterodimers of psoralen and thymine derivatives: properties, structure and stereochemistry, *Photobiochem. Photobiophys.,* 3, 113, 1981.
20. **deMol, N. J., Beijersbergen van Henegouwen, G. M. J., Mohn, G. R., Glickman, B. W., and van Kleef, P. M.,** On the involvement of singlet oxygen in mutation induction by 8-methoxypsoralen and UVA irradiation in *Escherichia coli* K12, *Mutat. Res.,* 82, 23, 1981.
21. **deMol, N. J. and Beijersbergen van Henegouwen, G. M. J.,** Relation between some photobiological properties of furocoumarins and their extent of singlet oxygen production, *Photochem. Photobiol.,* 33, 815, 1981.
22. **Magnus, I. A. and Young, A. R.,** Modification of photocarcinogenesis by 5-methoxypsoralen and sunscreens, in *Psoralens in Cosmetics and Dermatology,* Cahn, J., Forlot, P., Grupper, C., Meybeck, A., and Urbach, F., Eds., Pergamon Press, Elmsford, N.Y., 1981, 371.
23. **Kaidbey, K. H. and Kligman, A. M.,** Photosensitization by coumarin derivatives, *Arch. Dermatol.,* 117, 258, 1981.
24. **Ashwood-Smith, M. J., Poulton, G. A., and Liu, M.,** Photobiological activity of 5,7-dimethoxycoumarin, *Experientia,* 39, 262, 1983.
25. **Venturini, S., Tamaro, M., Monti-Bragadin, C., and Carlassare, F.,** Mutagenicity in *Salmonella typhimurium* of some angelicin derivatives proposed as new mono-functional agents for the photochemotherapy of psoriasis, *Mutat. Res.,* 88, 17, 1981.
26. **Shim, S. C., Ra, C. S., and Chae, K. H.,** Photocycloaddition of 5,7-dimethyoxycoumarin to 5-fluorouracil, *Bull. Kor. Chem. Soc.,* 1, 121, 1980 and *Chem. Abstr.,* 94, 93478r, 1981.
27. **Averbeck, D. and Moustacchi, E.,** Decreased photo-induced mutagenicity of mono-functional as opposed to bi-functional furocoumarins in yeast, *Photochem. Photobiol.,* 31, 475, 1980.
28. **Grossweiner, L. I. and Sherman, W. V.,** The effect of dark complexing on the photosensitized formation of 8-methoxypsoralen cross-links with DNA, *Photochem. Photobiol.,* 32, 697, 1980.

29. **Belogurov, A. A. and Zavilgelsky, G. B.,** Mutagenic effect of furocoumarin monoadducts and cross-links on bacteriophage lambda, *Mutat. Res.,* 84, 11, 1981.

30. **Dall'acqua, F., Vedaldi, D., Baccichetti, F., Bordin, F., and Averbeck, D.,** Photochemotherapy of skin-diseases: comparative studies on the photochemical and photobiological properties of various mono- and bi-functional agents, *Farmaco Ed. Sci.,* 36, 519, 1981.

31. **Grossweiner, L. I.,** Kinetics of furocoumarin photosensitization of DNA to near ultraviolet radiation, *Photochem. Photobiol.,* 34, 119, 1981.

32. **Bensasson, R. V., Salet, C., Land, E. J., and Rushton, F. A. P.,** Triplet excited state of the 4,5'-photoadduct of psoralen and thymine, *Photochem. Photobiol.,* 31, 129, 1980.

33. **Venturini, S., Tamaro, M., Monti-Bragadin, C., Bordin, F., Baccichetti, F., and Carlassare, F.,** Comparative mutagenicity of linear and angular furocoumarins in E. coli strains deficient in known repair functions, *Chem. Biol. Interact.,* 30, 203, 1980.

34. **Ashwood-Smith, M. J., Natarajan, A. T., and Poulton, G. A.,** Comparative photobiology of psoralens, in *Psoralens in Cosmetics and Dermatology,* Cahn, J., Forlot, P., Grupper, C., Meybeck, A., and Urbach, F., Eds., Pergamon Press, Elmsford, N.Y., 1981, 117.

35. **Rodighiero, G.,** Search for furocoumarin derivatives behaving as mono-functional reagents, in *Psoralens in Cosmetics and Dermatology,* Cahn, J., Forlot, P., Grupper, C., Meybeck, A., and Urbach, F., Eds., Pergamon Press, Elmsford, N.Y., 1981, 99.

36. **Lerman, S., Megaw, J., and Willis, I.,** The photoreactions of 8-methoxypsoralen with tryptophan and lens proteins, *Photochem. Photobiol.,* 31, 235, 1980.

37. **Allegri, G., Costa, C., DeAntoni, A., Baccichetti, F., and Vanzan, S.,** Effect of psoralen-induced photodermatitis on tryptophan metabolism in guinea pigs, *Farmaco Ed. Sci.,* 36, 557, 1981.

38. **DeAntoni, A., Costa, C., Allegri, G., Baccichetti, F., and Vanzan, S.,** Effect of psoralen-induced photodermatitis on tryptophan metabolism in rats, *Chem. Biol. Interact.,* 34, 11, 1981.

39. **Schmid, J., Brickl, R., Busch, U., and Koss, F. W.,** Comparison of pharmacokinetics, pharmacodynamics, and metabolism of 8-methoxypsoralen, 5-methoxypsoralen and 4,5',8-trimethylpsoralen, in *Psoralens in Cosmetics and Dermatology,* Cahn, J., Forlot, P., Grupper, C., Meybeck, A., and Urbach, F., Eds., Pergamon Press, Elmsford, N.Y., 1981, 109.

40. **Young, A. R. and Barth, J.,** Comparative studies on the photosensitizing potency of 5-methoxypsoralen and 8-methoxypsoralen as measured by cytolysis in *Paramecium caudatum* and *Tetrahymena pyriformis* and growth inhibition and survival in *Candida albicans, Photochem. Photobiol.,* 35, 83, 1982.

41. **Kagan, J. and Gabriel, R.,** *Candida utilis* as a convenient and safe substitute for the pathogenic yeast, *C. albicans* in Daniels' phototoxicity test, *Experientia,* 36, 587, 1980.

42. **Schimmer, O.,** Vergleich der photomutagenen Wirkungen von 5-MOP (Bergapten) und 8-MOP (Xanthotoxin) in *Chlamydomonas reinhardii, Mutat. Res.,* 89, 283, 1981.

43. **Ashwood-Smith, M. J., Poulton, G. A., Barker, M., and Mildenberger, M.,** 5-Methoxypsoralen, an ingredient in several suntan preparations, has lethal, mutagenic and clastogenic properties, *Nature (London),* 285, 407, 1980.

44. **Ashwood-Smith, M. J. and Poulton, G. A.,** Inappropriate regulations governing the use of oil of bergamot in suntan preparations, *Mutat. Res.,* 85, 389, 1981.

45. **Towers, G. H. N., Graham, E. A., Spenser, I. D., and Abramowski, Z.,** Phototoxic furanoquinolines of the *Rutaceae, Planta Med.,* 41, 136, 1981.

46. **Yasui, A., Winckler, K., and Laskowski, W.,** UV-induced reactivation and mutagenesis of λ-phages after treatment with 8-methoxypsoralen or thiopyronine and light, *Radiat. Environ. Biophys.,* 19, 239, 1981.

47. **Pani, B., Babudri, N., Venturini, S., Tamaro, M., Bordin, F., and Monti-Bragadin, C.,** Mutation induction and killing of prokaryotic and eukaryotic cells by 8-methoxypsoralen, 4,5'-dimethylangelicin, 5-methylangelicin, 4'-hydroxymethyl-4,5'-dimethylangelicin, *Teratogens, Carcinogens, Mutagens,* 1, 407, 1981.

48. **Yarosh, D. B., Johns, V., Mufti, S., Bernstein, C., and Bernstein, H.,** Inhibition of UV and psoralen-plus-light mutagenesis in phage T4 by gene 43 antimutator polymerase alleles, *Photochem. Photobiol.,* 31, 341, 1980.

49. **Wirth, H., Rauner, N., Gloor, M., Osswald, F., and Schnyder, U. W.,** On the influence of X-ray irradiation and photochemotherapy with 8-methoxypsoralen on the sebaceous gland of the Syrian hamster ear, *Dermatologica,* 162, 321, 1981.

50. **Natarajan, A. T., Verdegaal-Immerzeel, E. A. M., Ashwood-Smith, M. J., and Poulton, G. A.,** Chromosomal damage induced by furocoumarin and UVA in hamster and human cells including cells from patients with Ataxia telangiectasia and Xeroderma pigmentosum, *Mutat. Res.,* 84, 113, 1981.

51. **Ashwood-Smith, M. J., Natarajan, A. T., and Poulton, G. A.,** Comparative photobiology of psoralens, *J. Natl. Cancer Inst.,* 69, 189, 1982.

52. **Schenley, R. L. and Hsie, A. W.,** Interaction of 8-methoxypsoralen and near-UV light causes mutation and cytotoxicity in mammalian cells, *Photochem. Photobiol.,* 33, 179, 1981.

53. **Ljunggren, B., Bjellerup, M., and Carter, D. M.,** Dose-response relations in phototoxicity due to 8-methoxypsoralen and UV-A in man, *J. Invest. Dermatol.,* 76, 73, 1981.

54. **Cohen, L. F., Kraemer, K. H., Waters, H. L., Kohn, K. W., and Glaubiger, D. L.,** DNA crosslinking and cell survival in human lymphoid cells treated with 8-methoxypsoralen and long wavelength ultraviolet radiation, *Mutat. Res.,* 80, 347, 1981.

55. **Zajdela, F. and Bisagni, E.,** 5-Methoxypsoralen, the melanogenic additive in sun-tan preparations, is tumorigenic in mice exposed to 365 nm UV radiation, *Carcinogenesis,* 2, 121, 1981.

56. **VanderSluis, W. G., VanArkel, J., Fischer, F. C., and Labadie, R. P.,** Thin-layer chromatographic assay of photoactive compounds (furocoumarins) using the fungus *Penicillium expansum* as a test organism, *J. Chromatogr.,* 214, 349, 1981.

57. **Henriques, J. A. P. and Moustacchi, E.,** Sensitivity to photoaddition of mono- and bifunctional furocoumarins of X-ray sensitive mutants of *Saccharomyces cerevisiae, Photochem. Photobiol.,* 31, 557, 1980.

58. **Warren, R. A. J., Hudson, J. B., Downum, K., Graham, E. A., Norton, R., and Towers, G. H. N.,** Bacteriophages as indicators of the mechanism of action of photosensitizing agents, *Photobiochem. Photobiophys.,* 1, 385, 1980.

59. **Horio, T. and Watanabe, S.,** Photosensitization of *Trichophyton* with 8-methoxypsoralen to UV-A light radiation, *Br. J. Dermatol.,* 104, 397, 1981.

60. **Zaynoun, S. T., Aftimos, B. A., Tenekjian, K. K., and Kurban, A. K.,** Berloque dermatitis-a continuing cosmetic problem, *Contact Dermatitis,* 7, 111, 1981.

61. **Leick, V. and Nielsen, P. E.,** Photochemical effect of psoralens on TMV-RNA messenger activity in *in vitro* protein synthesis, *Photobiochem. Photobiophys.,* 2, 285, 1981.

62. **Veronese, F. M., Schiavon, O., Bevilacqua, R., Bordin, F., and Rodighiero, G.,** The effect of psoralens and angelicins on proteins in the presence of UV-A irradiation, *Photochem. Photobiol.,* 34, 351, 1981.

63. **Hearst, J. E.,** Psoralen photochemistry and nucleic acid structure. *J. Invest. Dermatol.,* 77, 39, 1981.

64. **Arnaud, R., Deflandre, A., Lang, G., and Lemaire, J.,** Propriétés photosensibilisatrices des furocoumarines. IV. Étude photochimique des furocoumarines methoxylées en solution aqueuse, *J. Chim. Phys.,* 78, 597, 1981.

65. **Arnaud, R., Deflandre, A., Malaval, A., Lang, G., and Lemaire, J.,** Propriétés photosensibilisatrices des furocoumarines. I. Photoreactivité des furocoumarines derivées du psoralène en presence d'ADN et de maléimide, *J. Chim. Phys.,* 76, 1133, 1979.

66. **Wat, C.-K., MacRae, W. D., Yamamoto, E., Towers, G. H. N., and Lam, J.,** Phototoxic effects of naturally occurring polyacetylenes and α-terthienyl on human erythrocytes, *Photochem. Photobiol.,* 32, 167, 1980.

67. **Arnason, T., Wat, C.-K., Downum, K., Yamamoto, E., Graham, E., and Towers, G. H. N.,** Photosensitization of *Escherichia coli* and *Saccharomyces cerevisiae* by phenylheptatriyne from *Bidens pilosa, Can. J. Microbiol.,* 26, 698, 1980.

68. **MacRae, W. D., Chan, G. F. Q., Wat, C.-K., Towers, G. H. N., and Lam, J.,** Examination of naturally occurring polyacetylenes and α-terthienyl for their ability to induce cytogenetic damage, *Experientia,* 36, 1096, 1980.

69. **Arnason, T., Swain, T., Wat, C.-K., Graham, E. A., Partington, S., Towers, G. H. N., and Lam, J.,** Mosquito larvicidal activity of polyacetylenes from species in the *Asteraceae, Biochem. Syst. Ecol.,* 9, 63, 1981.

70. **Arnason, T., Chan, G. F. Q., Wat, C.-K., Downum, K., and Towers, G. H. N.,** Oxygen requirement for near-UV mediated cytotoxicity of α-terthienyl to *Escherichia coli* and *Saccharomyces cerevisiae, Photochem. Photobiol.,* 33, 821, 1981.

71. **Gommers, F. J., Bakker, J., and Smits, L.,** Effects of singlet oxygen generated by the nematicidal compound α-terthienyl from *Tagetes* on the nematode *Aphelenchus avenae, Nematologica,* 26, 369, 1980.

72. **Bakker, J., Gommers, F. J., Nieuwenhuis, I., and Wynberg, H.,** Photoactivation of the nematicidal compound α-terthienyl from the roots of marigolds (*Tagetes* species). A possible singlet oxygen role, *J. Biol. Chem.,* 254, 1841, 1979.

73. **Kagan, J., Gabriel, R., and Singh, S. P.,** 1,4-Diphenylbutadiyne, a new non-photodynamic phototoxic compound, *Photochem. Photobiol.,* 32, 607, 1980.

74. **Kagan, J., Gabriel, R., and Reed, S. A.,** Alpha-terthienyl, a non-photodynamic phototoxic compound, *Photochem. Photobiol.,* 31, 465, 1980.

75. **Wat, C.-K., Prasad, S. K., Graham, E. A., Partington, S., Arnason, T., Towers, G. H. N., and Lam, J.,** Photosensitization of invertebrates by natural polyacetylenes, *Biochem. Syst. Ecol.,* 9, 59, 1981.

76. **Pfyffer, G. E., Panfil, I., and Towers, G. H. N.,** Monofunctional covalent photobinding of dictamnine, a furoquinoline alkaloid, to DNA as target *in vitro, Photochem. Photobiol.,* 35, 63, 1982.

77. **Towers, G. H. N., Whitehead, F. W., Abramowski, Z. A., and Mitchell, J. C.,** Dictamnine, an alkaloid which crosslinks DNA in the presence of ultraviolet light, *Biochem. Biophys. Res. Commun.,* 95, 603, 1980.

78. **Ashwood-Smith, M. J., Towers, G. H. N., Abramowski, Z., Poulton, G. A., and Liu, M.,** Photobiological studies with dictamnine, a furoquinoline alkaloid, *Mutat. Res.*, 102, 401, 1982.

79. **Wagner, S., Feldman, A., and Snipes, W.,** Recovery from damage induced by acridine plus nearultraviolet light in *Escherichia coli*, *Photochem. Photobiol.*, 35, 73, 1982.

80. **Wagner, S., Taylor, W. D., Keith, A., and Snipes, W.,** Effects of acridine plus near-ultraviolet light on *Escherichia coli* membranes and DNA *in vivo*, *Photochem. Photobiol.*, 32, 771, 1980.

81. **Chahidi, C., Aubailly, M., Momzikoff, A., Bazin, M., and Santus, R.,** Photophysical and photosensitizing properties of 2-amino-4-pteridinone: a natural pigment, *Photochem. Photobiol.*, 33, 641, 1981.

82. **Santus, R., Momzikoff, A., and Salet, C., in** *Proceedings of the International Conference on Oxygen and Oxy-Radicals in Chemistry and Biology*, Academic Press, New York, 1981.

83. **Snipes, W., Keller, G., Woog, J., Vickroy, T., Deering, R., and Keith, A.,** Inactivation of lipid-containing viruses by hydrophobic sensitizers and near ultraviolet radiation, *Photochem. Photobiol.*, 29, 785, 1979.

Chapter 10

CARCINOGENS IN EDIBLE MUSHROOMS

Bela Toth

TABLE OF CONTENTS

I. INTRODUCTION

In early 1974, our research activity focused on hydrazines occurring in edible mushrooms. Prior to this we conducted a series of investigations with hydrazines synthesized for medical, industrial, and agricultural use.[1,2] The results of these investigations proved that most chemicals of this class are cancer-inducing substances in laboratory animals. Since 1974 it became evident that these naturally occurring hydrazine ingredients of edible mushrooms are also carcinogenic in animals.[3-13] The mushroom species are as follows.

A. *Agaricus bisporus*

The commonly eaten cultivated mushroom of commerce in the Western hemisphere, *A. bisporus* (Figure 1) belongs to the Agaricaceae family, the meadow mushrooms. *A. bisporus* was in reality derived from several different species and its continual propagation over several centuries has resulted in several commercial strains which have no exact counterpart in nature. *Agaricus campestris*, commonly known as the "pink bottom", is probably the most closely related of any of the common species encountered in North America.[14] *A. bisporus* is usually eaten cooked, although some people prefer it raw. Approximately 280 million kg of this fungus was consumed (through production and import) in the U.S. in 1982.[15] The annual production in other leading countries, according to 1972 figures in millions of kilograms, was France, 113; Taiwan, 84; U.K., 45; Netherlands, 39; Italy, 30; Federal Republic of Germany, 27.[16]

B. *Gyromitra esculenta*

G. esculenta (Figure 2) is one of the false morel mushrooms. In addition to *Gyromitra*, the group includes *Helvella* and related species for a total of 11,[14] and is a highly varied group, with toxic and edible species resembling each other closely enough to be confused. Of the entire group, only one specimen, the *Gyromitra esculenta*, has been studied in depth and is an often-sought, delicious mushroom, although occasionally some problems have arisen after its consumption. For example, in certain instances, people have died after ingesting the mushroom, while more often illness followed and people were affected to various degrees.[17] Precise information on the consumption of false morel mushrooms is not available, but it is estimated that at least 1 million people in the world eat this fungus yearly.[17] According to an expert, 100,000 persons annually consume *Gyromitra esculenta* in the U.S. alone.[18] A knowledgeable investigator believes that hundreds of thousands of Finns enjoy this mushroom every spring[19] and a considerable amount of false morel consumption was reported in Germany, particularly between World Wars I and II.[20]

In the following, the results of chemical and carcinogenesis investigations of hydrazines and related compounds occurring in *Agaricus bisporus* and *Gyromitra esculenta* are described in detail.

II. *AGARICUS BISPORUS*

A. Chemistry

In 1960, a hydrazide β-N-[γ-L(+)glutamyl]-4-hydroxymethylphenylhydrazine, synonym agaritine, was identified in this fungus in amounts up to 0.04% based on fresh tissue weight.[21] Subsequently, the mushrooms bought in local food stores were found to contain between 0.04 and 0.07% agaritine.[22] The mushrooms kept in storage in a refrigerator lost the agaritine content between 2 and 47% in the first week and between 36 and 76% in the second week. Canned mushrooms did not contain any detectable agaritine, while the frozen fungus contained 0.033% and the cooked one lost only 32% of its original agaritine content. After administration by gavage agaritine reached all parts of the GI tract of the mouse in 15 min and was not detectable after 3 hr.[22] The mammalian enzyme γ-glutamyltranspeptidase was

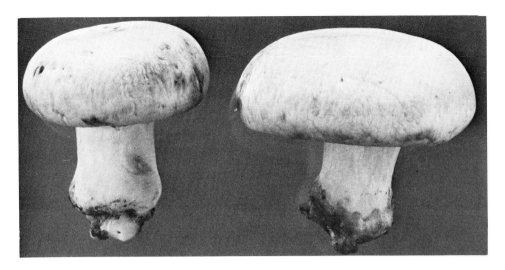

FIGURE 1.   The cultivated mushroom of commerce in the Western hemisphere, *Agaricus bisporus.*

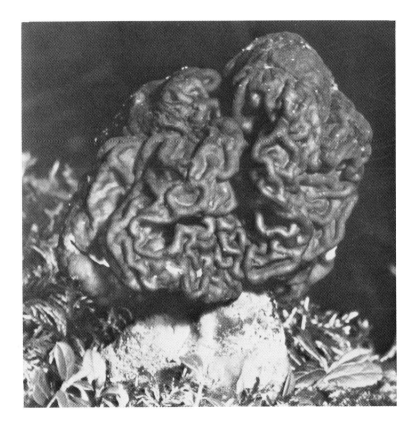

FIGURE 2.   One of the false morel mushrooms, *Gyromitra esculenta.*

found capable of splitting agaritine to glutamic acid and 4-(hydroxymethyl)phenyl-hydrazine.[23] Furthermore, 4-(hydroxymethyl)phenylhydrazine in vitro with lithium alumi-num hydride in boiling ether undergoes further changes and yields through an intermediate 4-methylphenylhydrazine.[24] Finally, 4-(hydroxymethyl)benzenediazonium ion was detected at 0.6 ppm level in *A. bisporus,* which is apparently the hydrolytic product of agaritine (Figure 3).[25]

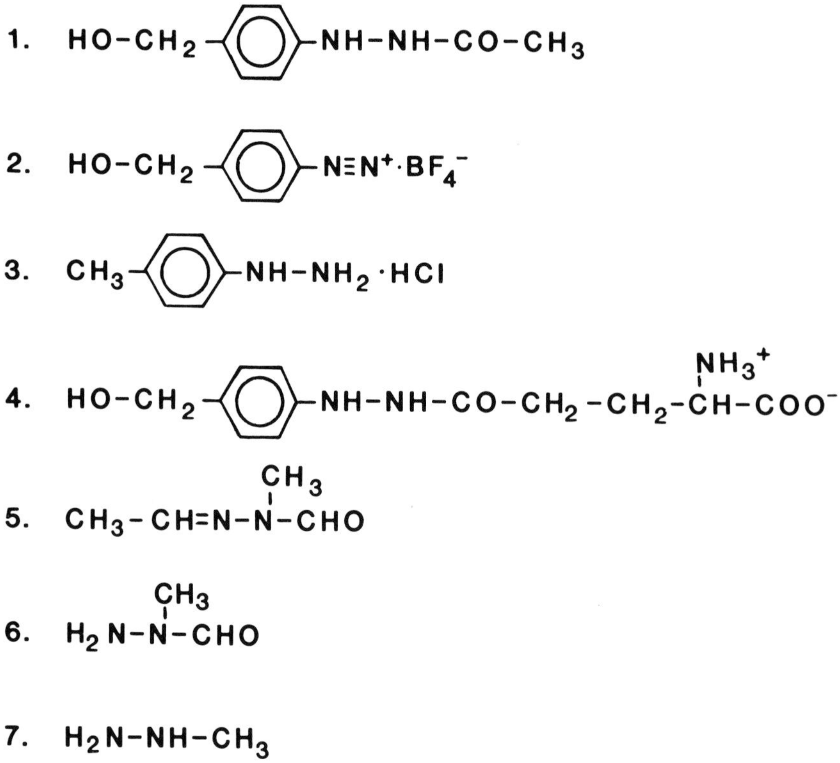

1.   HO–CH$_2$–⟨○⟩–NH–NH–CO–CH$_3$

2.   HO–CH$_2$–⟨○⟩–N≡N$^+$·BF$_4^-$

3.   CH$_3$–⟨○⟩–NH–NH$_2$·HCl

4.   HO–CH$_2$–⟨○⟩–NH–NH–CO–CH$_2$–CH$_2$–CH–COO$^-$ with NH$_3^+$ on the CH

5.   CH$_3$–CH=N–N–CHO with CH$_3$ substituent

6.   H$_2$N–N–CHO with CH$_3$ substituent

7.   H$_2$N–NH–CH$_3$

FIGURE 3.   Chemical structures of: (1) *N'*-acetyl-4-(hydroxymethylphenyl)hydrazine; (2) 4-(hydroxymethyl)benzenediazonium tetrafluoroborate; (3) 4-methylphenylhydrazine hydrochloride; (4) agaritine; (5) gyromitrin; (6) *N*-methyl-*N*-formylhydrazine, and (7) methylhydrazine.

B. Carcinogenesis

The *N'*-acetyl derivative of 4-hydroxymethylphenylhydrazine, an enzymatic product of agaritine, was synthesized at this institute. This compound was found to be stable in tap water, therefore it was administered as a 0.0625% solution in the drinking water for the life span of Swiss albino mice. Compared with that in untreated controls, the lung tumor incidence rose in treated animals from 15 to 35% in females and from 22 to 48% in males, whereas the incidence of blood vessel tumors increased from 8 to 32% in females and from 5 to 30% in males.[26,27]

4-Hydroxymethylphenylhydrazine was also reported to yield under special conditions to 4-methylphenylhydrazine (4-MPH).[24] Since this compound was commercially available and its hydrochloride form was stable enough, another long-term carcinogenesis experiment was set up. The hydrochloride form of 4-MPH was administered as 10 weekly s.c. injections of 140 µg/g body weight and as 7 weekly intragastric instillations of 250 µg/g body weight in physiological saline to Swiss mice. The treatment given s.c. resulted in induction of lung tumors in incidences of 36% in females and 44% in males, while intragastric treatment caused a 40% incidence in females. In addition, it gave rise to blood vessel tumors by the intragastric route in incidences of 32% in females and 18% in males.[28,29]

4-Methylphenylhydrazine hydrochloride (4-MPH) was also administered to randomly bred Swiss mice as 26 weekly s.c. injections of 140 µg/g of body weight and *N'*-acetyl-4-(hydroxymethyl)phenylhydrazine (AMPH) as 26 weekly s.c. injections of 500 µg/g. As a solvent control, physiological saline was also given as 26 weekly s.c. injections of 0.01 mℓ/g. The 4-MPH-treatment induced a significant incidence (24%) of fibrosarcomas in males. In the 4-MPH-treated females and some AMPH-treated male mice, a few soft-tissue tumors were observed, however, their appearance could not be related to treatment.[30,31]

Table 1
TUMOR SPECTRA OF MUSHROOM HYDRAZINES AND RELATED CHEMICALS

No.	Mushroom	Chemical	Species	Target organs
1	*Agaricus bisporus*	N′-Acetyl-4-(hydroxymethyl)phenylhydrazine	Mice	Lungs, blood vessels
2	*Agaricus bisporus*	4-(Hydroxymethyl)benzenediazonium tetrafluoroborate	Mice	Glandular stomach, skin, subcutis
3	*Agaricus bisporus*	4-Methylphenylhydrazine hydrochloride	Mice	Lungs, blood vessels, subcutis
4	*Agaricus bisporus*	Agaritine	Mice	—
5	*Gyromitra esculenta*	Gyromitrin	Mice	Lungs, preputial glands, clitoral glands, forestomach
6	*Gyromitra esculenta*	N-Methyl-N-formylhydrazine	Mice	Lungs, liver, gallbladder, bile ducts, blood vessels
			Hamsters	Liver, bile ducts, gallbladder, Kupffer cells
7	*Gyromitra esculenta*	Methylhydrazine	Mice	Lungs
			Hamsters	Kupffer cells, cecum

The 4-(hydroxymethyl)benzenediazonium ion is present in the extracts of *Agaricus bisporus*.[25] The tetrafluoroborate salt was synthesized in this institute and was given as 26 weekly s.c. injections at 50 μg/g body weight to Swiss mice. The treatment induced tumors in the subcutis and skin at incidences of 20 and 12%, respectively.[32-34]

4-(Hydroxymethyl)benzenediazonium tetrafluoroborate was also administered as a single intragastric instillation at 400 μg/g body weight basis to Swiss albino mice. The treatment gave rise to glandular stomach tumors at incidences of 30% in females and 32% in males. Histopathologically, the tumors were classified as polypoid adenomas and adenocarcinomas.[35-37]

Since the synthesis of agaritine required the development of new techniques, the initiation of the chronic experiment with agaritine was delayed.[35] This chemical was administered as a 0.0625% solution in drinking water for life to Swiss mice. In addition, because the dose was too toxic for the males, another 50 male mice were given a 0.03125% solution of the compound. Consumption of the chemical resulted in no detectable carcinogenic action under the experimental conditions. During the course of the experiment, however, a substantial number of animals developed convulsive seizures (Table 1).[38-40]

C. Mutagenesis
Some of these compounds were also studied for and showed mutagenic activities in bacterial and mammalian cell systems.[41,42]

III. *GYROMITRA ESCULENTA*

A. Chemistry
Of the eleven *Gyromitras* and related species, only *Gyromitra esculenta* was analyzed chemically for hydrazine compounds. The types and amounts of hydrazine derivatives found in this fungus are listed below:[43-47]

Acetaldehyde methylformylhydrazone (MFHO)	49.9 mg/kg
Propanal MFHO	1.0 mg/kg
Butanal MFHO	0.6 mg/kg
3-Methylbutanal MFHO	2.2 mg/kg
Pentanal MFHO	0.8 mg/kg
Hexanal MFHO	1.4 mg/kg
Octanal MFHO	0.2 mg/kg
trans-2-Octenal MFHO	0.6 mg/kg
cis-2-Octenal MFHO	0.3 mg/kg
N-Methyl-N-formylhydrazine (MFH) (by dry weight)	500 mg/kg
Methylhydrazine	14 mg/kg

N-Methyl-N-formylhydrazine was postulated as a hydrolysis product of gyromitrin.[48] Later, gyromitrin at 37°C under different acidic conditions (pH 1 to 2) that mimic the milieu of human stomach is converted through the intermediate N-methyl-N-formylhydrazine to methylhydrazine. In addition, methylhydrazine is formed in the mouse stomach after oral administration of gyromitrin (Figure 3).[49,50]

The false morel mushroom *Gyromitra esculenta* was collected in Ontario, Canada and analyzed in this laboratory. It was found to contain concentrations of G similar to those reported by the Finnish investigators.[51]

We also analyzed canned *Gyromitra esculenta* from Switzerland and found MH at levels of 2 to 3 μg/g in the flesh and 11 μg/mℓ in the juice.[51]

The toxic action of methylhydrazine was prevented in mice by pyridoxine hydrochloride. The toxic symptoms caused by N-methyl-N-formylhydrazine were, however, only slightly inhibited by this vitamin.[52]

B. Carcinogenesis

Methylhydrazine (MH) sulfate was administered as a 0.001% solution in drinking water for the life span of Swiss mice from 6 weeks of age. In the treated females and males, the lung tumor incidences were 46 and 46%, respectively.[53-55]

MH was also administered as a 0.01% solution in the drinking water of 6-week-old hamsters for the remainder of their life. The treatment gave rise to malignant histiocytomas and tumors of the cecum. Almost one third (32%) of the females and 54% of the males developed malignant histiocytomas, whereas the incidence of tumors of the cecum was 18% in females and 14% in males.[56-58]

Continuous administration of 0.0078% of N-methyl-N-formylhydrazine (MFH) in drinking water for life to 6-week-old Swiss mice produced tumors of the liver, lungs, gall bladder, and bile duct. The tumor incidences in these four tissues in females were 44, 60, 8, and 4%, respectively, whereas in males they were 22, 40, 10, and 10%, respectively. The higher dose of 0.0156%, given under identical conditions, had no tumorigenic effect since it proved too toxic for the animals.[59-61] The compound was also given as a 0.0039% solution under conditions similar to those above. It induced tumors of the lungs, liver, blood vessels, gall bladder, and bile ducts of mice. The tumor incidences in these five tissues in females were, respectively, 86, 36, 34, 10, and 2%, while in the males they were 68, 56, 8, 10, and 12%, respectively.[62,63] Two additional lower dose levels of 0.002 and 0.001% MFH were also administered under conditions identical to those in the Swiss mice. The treatment induced lung, blood vessel, liver, and gall bladder tumors. The 0.002% solution gave rise to tumors of the above tissues at incidences of 94, 40, 0, and 6% in females and 62, 14, 28, and 16% in males, respectively. The 0.001% solution also gave rise to the same tumor types in the following incidences: 78, 20, 2, and 0% in females and 72, 26, 12, and 12% in males.[64,65] Finally the compound was administered at 0.0005 and 0.00025% dose levels under conditions similar to those in Swiss mice. At the high dose level, 64% of the females and 48% of the males developed lung tumors while the corresponding tumor incidences at the lower dose level were 62% in the females and 54% in the males.[66-68]

MFH was also given as a 0.0078% solution in drinking water to hamsters for life from 6 weeks of age. The treatment gave rise to liver cell tumors, malignant histiocytomas, and tumors of the gall bladder and bile ducts. The tumor incidences in these four tissues were 38, 48, 6, and 2% in females and 48, 20, 16, and 14% in males, respectively.[69,70]

In another study single injections of MFH were given to Swiss mice. The females received 180 μg MFH/g body weight, while two groups of males were treated either with 120 or 100 μg MFH/g body weight. The treatment resulted in lung tumor induction at an incidence of 40% in the females. In males treated with the higher and lower doses, the incidences of preputial gland tumors were 12 and 12%, respectively.[71]

Acetaldehyde methylformylhydrazone (gyromitrin) was administered in 52 repeated weekly intragastric instillations at 100 μg/g body weight. The treatment gave rise to tumors of the lungs, preputial glands, forestomach, and clitoral glands. The tumor incidences in these four tissues in treated females were 70, 0, 16, and 12%, respectively, whereas in the treated males they were 40, 90, 0, and 0%.[72,73]

Gyromitrin was also given in another experiment to mice in 12 repeated weekly s.c. injections on the basis of 50 μg/g body weight. The treatment induced lung and preputial gland tumors at incidences of 51 and 0% in females and 46 and 28% in males, respectively (Table 1).[74]

C. Mutagenesis

Some of these mushroom hydrazines exhibited mutagenic activities in bacterial and mammalian cell systems.[41,42]

IV. CONCLUSION

Chemical and carcinogenesis investigations have been conducted with a series of hydrazines and related chemical ingredients of the cultivated mushroom of commerce, *Agaricus bisporus*, and one of the wild and edible false morel mushrooms, *Gyromitra esculenta*. Two chemical constituents of *Agaricus bisporus* induced tumors in five tissues of mice and three compound ingredients of *Gyromitra esculenta* gave rise to tumors in nine tissues of mice and hamsters.

In view of these findings and because the population consumes substantial amounts of *Agaricus bisporus* and, to a much smaller extent, *Gyromitra esculenta*, further research, particularly in the fields of carcinogenesis, chemistry, and human epidemiology, is highly recommended.

REFERENCES

1. **Toth, B.,** Synthetic and naturally occurring hydrazines as possible cancer causative agents, *Cancer Res.,* 35, 3693, 1975.
2. **Toth, B.,** Actual new cancer-causing hydrazines, hydrazides and hydrazones, *J. Cancer Res. Clin. Oncol.,* 97, 97, 1980.
3. **Schmeltz, I., Hoffmann, D., and Toth, B.,** Hydrazines: occurrence, analysis and carcinogenic activity as related to structure, *Proceedings of the Symposium on Structural Correlates of Carcinogenesis and Mutagenesis. A Guide to Testing Priorities?* FDA/OS, Washington, D.C., 172, 1977.
4. **Toth, B.,** The large bowel carcinogenic effects of hydrazines and related compounds occurring in nature and in the environment, *Cancer,* 40(Suppl.), 2427, 1977.
5. **Toth, B.,** Additional series of carcinogenic hydrazines, 12th Int. Cancer Congr., Buenos Aires, 1, 30, 1978.
6. **Toth, B.,** Hepatocarcinogenesis by hydrazine mycotoxins of edible mushrooms, *J. Toxicol. Environ. Health,* 5, 193, 1979.
7. **Toth, B. and Nagel, D.,** Carcinogenesis by edible mushroom hydrazines, *Proc. Am. Assoc. Cancer Res.,* 20, 43, 1979.
8. **Toth, B.,** Mushroom hydrazines: occurrence, metabolism, carcinogenesis and environmental implications, in *Naturally Occurring Carcinogens-Mutagens and Modulators of Carcinogenesis,* Miller, E. C. et al., Eds., University Park Press, Baltimore, 1979, 57.
9. **Toth, B.,** Carcinogenesis by mushroom hydrazines, in *Biology of the Cancer Cell,* Proc. 5th Meet. Eur. Assoc. Cancer Res., Vienna, Austria, 53, 1980.

10. **Toth, B.,** Carcinogenesis by mushroom hydrazines. Additional investigations with naturally occurring mycotoxins, in *Biology of the Cancer Cell,* Proc. 5th Meet. Eur. Assoc. Cancer Res., Vienna, Austria, 45, 1980.

11. **Toth, B. and Ross, A.,** Cultivated mushroom mycotoxins: carcinogenesis and chemistry, Proc. 6th Meet. Eur. Assoc. Cancer Res., Budapest, Hungary, 166, 1981.

12. **Toth, B.,** Hydrazines and related compounds in colonic carcinogenesis. Falk Symposium, Titisee, Germany, in *Colonic Carcinogenesis,* Malt, R. A. and Williamson, R. C. N., Eds., MTP Press, Lancaster, England, 1982, 165.

13. **Toth, B.,** Mushroom hydrazines and diazonium ions: carcinogenesis, mutagenesis and chemistry, in *Proc. 13th Int. Cancer Congr.,* Seattle, Washington, 66, 1982.

14. **Miller, O. K.,** *Mushrooms of North America,* E. P. Dutton, New York, 1972.

15. U.S. Department of Agriculture, Statistical Reporting Science, Crop Reporting Board, *Mushrooms, Vg 2-1-2,* Washington, D.C., 1982, 1.

16. **Maw, G. A. and Flegg, P. B.,** The mushrooms as a source of dietary protein, in *Glasshouse Crop Annual Report,* Littlehampton, England, 1974, 137.

17. **Simmons, D. M.,** The mushroom toxins, *Del. Med. J.,* 43, 177, 1971.

18. **Miller, O. K.,** Personal communication, 1976.

19. **Pyysalo, H.,** Tests for gyromitrin, a poisonous compound in false morel *Gyromitra esculenta, Z. Lebensm. Unters. Forsch.,* 160, 325, 1976.

20. **Franke, S., Freimuth, U. and List, P. H.,** Über die Giftigkeit der Frühjahrslorchel *Gyromitra (Helvella) esculenta, Fr. Arch. Toxicol.,* 22, 293, 1967.

21. **Levenberg, B.,** Structure and enzymatic cleavage of agaritine, a new phenylhydrazide of L-glutamic acid isolated from agaricaceae, *J. Am. Chem. Soc.,* 83, 503, 1960.

22. **Ross, A., Nagel, D. L., and Toth, B.,** Occurrence, stability and decomposition of β-N[γ-L(+)-glutamyl]-4-hydroxymethylphenylhydrazine (agaritine) from the mushroom *Agaricus bisporus, J. Food Chem. Toxicol.,* 20, 903, 1982.

23. **Gigliotti, H.,** Studies on the γ-Glutamyltransferase and Arylhydrazine Oxidase Activities of *Agaricus bisporus,* Ph.D. dissertation, University of Michigan, Ann Arbor, 1963.

24. **Gigliotti, H. and Levenberg, H.,** Studies on the γ-glutamyltransferase of *Agaricus bisporus, J. Biol. Chem.,* 239, 2274, 1964.

25. **Ross, A. E., Nagel, D., and Toth, B.,** Evidence for the occurrence and formation of diazonium ions in the *Agaricus bisporus* mushroom and its extracts, *J. Agric. Food Chem.,* 30, 521, 1982.

26. **Toth, B. and Nagel, D.,** Tumorigenicity of the N′-acetyl derivative of 4-hydroxymethylphenylhydrazine, an ingredient of *Agaricus bisporus, Proc. Am. Assoc. Cancer Res.,* 18, 15, 1977.

27. **Toth, B., Nagel, D., Patil, K., Erickson, J., and Antonson, K.,** Tumor induction with the N′-acetyl derivative of 4-hydroxymethylphenylhydrazine, a metabolite of agaritine of *Agaricus bisporus, Cancer Res.,* 38, 177, 1978.

28. **Toth, B., Tompa, A., and Patil, K.,** Tumorigenic effect of 4-methylphenylhydrazine hydrochloride in Swiss mice, *Z. Krebsforsch. Klin. Onkol.,* 89, 245, 1977.

29. **Toth, B. and Jae, H. S.,** Carcinogenesis and chemistry of mycotoxins and related compounds of *Agaricus bisporus, Proc. Am. Assoc. Cancer Res.,* 22, 114, 1981.

30. **Toth, B.,** Tumorigenesis with 4-methylphenylhydrazine hydrochloride in mice, *Fed. Proc. Fed. Am. Soc. Exp. Biol.,* 36, 1987, 1977.

31. **Toth, B. and Nagel, D.,** Studies on the tumorigenic potential of 4-substituted phenylhydrazines by subcutaneous route, *J. Toxicol. Environ. Health,* 8, 1, 1981.

32. **Toth, B., Nagel, D., and Ross, A.,** Occurrence and the carcinogenic action of 4-(hydroxymethyl)benzenediazonium ion (4-HMBD), *Proc. Am. Assoc. Cancer Res.,* 21, 73, 1980.

33. **Toth, B., Patil, K., and Jae, H. S.,** Carcinogenesis of 4-(hydroxymethyl)benzenediazonium ion (tetrafluoroborate) of *Agaricus bisporus, Cancer Res.,* 41, 2444, 1981.

34. **Toth, B. and Nagel, D.,** Carcinogenesis by mycotoxins of two edible mushrooms, *Lab. Invest.,* 44, 67A, 1981.

35. **Wallcave, L., Nagel, D., Raha, C. R., Jae, H. S., Bronczyk, S., Kupper, R., and Toth, B.,** An improved synthesis of agaritine, *J. Org. Chem.,* 44, 3752, 1979.

36. **Toth, B., Nagel, D., and Ross, A.,** Gastric tumorigenesis by a single dose of 4-(hydroxymethyl)benzenediazonium ion of *Agaricus bisporus, Br. J. Cancer,* 46, 417, 1982.

37. **Toth, B.,** Gastric carcinogenesis by 4-(hydroxymethyl)benzenediazonium ion (tetrafluoroborate) of *Agaricus bisporus, Proc. Am. Assoc. Cancer Res.,* 23, 50, 1982.

38. **Toth, B., Nagel, D., Shimizu, H., Sornson, H., Issenberg, P., and Erickson, J.,** Tumorigenicity of *n*-propyl-, *n*-amyl and allyl-hydrazines. Toxicity of agaritine, *Proc. Am. Assoc. Cancer Res.,* 16, 61, 1975.

39. **Toth, B., Shimizu, H., Sornson, H., Issenberg, P., and Erickson, J.,** Sex dependent toxicity of four chemicals, *Res. Commun. Chem. Pathol. Pharmacol.,* 10, 577, 1975.

40. **Toth, B., Raha, C. R., Wallcave, L., and Nagel, D.,** Attempted tumor induction with agaritine in mice, *Anticancer Res.,* 1, 255, 1981.
41. **Kuszynski, C., Langenbach, R., Malick, L., Tompa, A., and Toth, B.,** Liver cell-mediated mutagenesis of V-79 cells by hydrazine and related compounds, *Environ. Mutagenesis,* 3, 323, 1981.
42. **Rogan, E. G., Walker, B. A., Gingell, R., Nagel, D., and Toth, B.,** Microbial mutagenicity of selected hydrazines, *Mutat. Res.,* 102, 413, 1982.
43. **Schmidlin-Mészáros, J.,** Gyromitrin in Trockenlorcheln (Gyromitra esculenta sicc), *Mitt. Geb. Lebensmittelunters. Hyg.,* 65, 453, 1975.
44. **Pyysalo, H. and Niskanen, A.,** On the occurrence of N-methyl-N-formylhydrazones in fresh and processed false morel, *Gyromitra esculenta, J. Agric. Food Chem.,* 25, 644, 1977.
45. **Pyysalo, H. and Honkanen, E.,** Mass spectra of some N-methyl-N-formylhydrazines, *Acta Chem. Scand.,* 30, 792, 1976.
46. **Pyysalo, H.,** Some new toxic compounds in the false morels, *Gyromitra esculenta, Naturwissenschaften,* 62, 395, 1975.
47. **List, P. H. and Luft, P.,** Gyromitrin, das Gift der Frühjahrslorchel *Helvella (Gyromitra) esculenta, Z. Pilzkd.,* 34, 3, 1968.
48. **List, P. H. and Luft, P.,** Gyromitrin das Gift der Frühjahrslorchel, *Arch. Pharmacol.,* 301, 294, 1968.
49. **Nagel, D., Toth, B., and Kupper, R.,** Formation of methylhydrazine from acetaldehyde N-methyl-N-formylhydrazone of *Gyromitra esculenta, Proc. Am. Assoc. Cancer Res.,* 17, 9, 1976.
50. **Nagel, D., Wallcave, L., Toth, B., and Kupper, R.,** Formation of methylhydrazine from acetalhyde N-methyl-N-formylhydrazone, a component of *Gyromitra esculenta, Cancer Res.,* 37, 3458, 1977.
51. **Wallcave, L.,** unpublished data, 1978.
52. **Toth, B. and Erickson, J.,** Reversal of the toxicity of hydrazines analogues by pyridoxine hydrochloride, *Toxicology,* 7, 31, 1977.
53. **Toth, B.,** Hydrazine, methylhydrazine and methylhydrazine sulfate carcinogenesis in Swiss mice. Failure of ammonium hydroxide to interfere in the development of tumors, *Int. J. Cancer,* 9, 109, 1972.
54. **Toth, B., Shimizu, H., Nagel, D., and Somogyi, A.,** Tumorigenesis studies with hydrazine derivatives. II. *Meet. Eur. Assoc. Cancer Res.,* Heidelberg, Germany, 36, 1973.
55. **Toth, B. and Nagel, D.,** Structure activity studies with methylated hydrazines in tumorigenesis, *Fed. Proc. Fed. Am. Soc. Exp. Biol.,* 35, 409, 1976.
56. **Toth, B. and Shimizu, H.,** Malignant histiocytoma induction by methylhydrazine in golden hamsters. Histologic and ultrastructural findings, *Sci. Proc. Am. Assoc. Pathol. Bacteriol.,* 70, 10a, 1973.
57. **Toth, B. and Shimizu, H.,** Methylhydrazine tumorigenesis in Syrian golden hamsters and the morphology of malignant histiocytomas, *Cancer Res.,* 33, 2744, 1973.
58. **Toth, B., Shimizu, H., and Nagel, D.,** Tumorigenic hydrazine compounds, 11th Int. Cancer Congr., Florence, Italy, 2, 37, 1974.
59. **Toth, B. and Nagel, D.,** Cancer induction with N-methyl-N-formylhydrazine, an ingredient of the false morel, 2nd Int. Mycol. Congr., Tampa, Fla., 2, 674, 1977.
60. **Toth, B.,** Tumor induction studies with hydrazine derivative ingredients of mushrooms, *Agaricus bisporus and Gyromitra esculenta,* 4th Meet. Eur. Assoc. Cancer Res., Lyon, France, 68, 1977.
61. **Toth, B. and Nagel, D.,** Tumors induced in mice by N-methyl-N-formylhydrazine of the false morel *Gyromitra esculenta, J. Natl. Cancer Inst.,* 60, 201, 1978.
62. **Toth, B. and Nagel, D.,** Mushroom toxin: N-methyl-N-formylhydrazine carcinogenesis in mice, *Proc. Am. Assoc. Cancer Res.,* 19, 42, 1978.
63. **Toth, B., Patil, K., Erickson, J., and Kupper, R.,** False morel mushroom *Gyromitra esculenta* toxin: N-methyl-N-formylhydrazine carcinogenesis in mice, *Mycopathologia,* 68, 121, 1979.
64. **Toth, B. and Nagel, D.,** Investigations on the carcinogenicity of hydrazine mycotoxins of an edible mushroom, *Fed. Proc. Fed. Am. Soc. Exp. Biol.,* 38, 1450, 1979.
65. **Toth, B. and Patil, K.,** The tumorigenic effect of low dose levels of N-methyl-N-formylhydrazine in mice, *Neoplasma,* 27, 25, 1980.
66. **Toth, B.,** Influence of chain length on N-alkyl-N-formylhydrazine carcinogenesis, *Fed. Proc. Fed. Am. Soc. Exp. Biol.,* 40, 746, 1981.
67. **Toth, B.,** Dose response studies in carcinogenesis by N-methyl-N-formylhydrazine of *Gyromitra esculenta, Lab. Invest.,* 46, 83A, 1982.
68. **Toth, B. and Patil, K.,** Tumorigenicity of minute dose levels of N-methyl-N-formylhydrazine of *Gyromitra esculenta, Mycopathologia,* 78, 11, 1982.
69. **Toth, B. and Nagel, D.,** Carcinogenesis in the Syrian golden hamster by N-methyl-N-formylhydrazine (MFH) of the false morel mushroom, *Fed. Proc. Fed. Am. Soc. Exp. Biol.,* 37, 231, 1978.
70. **Toth, B. and Patil, K.,** Carcinogenic effects in the Syrian golden hamster of N-methyl-N-formylhydrazine of the false morel mushroom *Gyromitra esculenta, J. Cancer Res. Clin. Oncol.,* 93, 109, 1979.
71. **Toth, B. and Patil, K.,** Carcinogenesis by a single dose of N-methyl-N-formylhydrazine, *J. Toxicol. Environ. Health,* 6, 577, 1980.

72. **Toth, B.,** Carcinogenesis by gyromitrin of *Gyromitra esculenta, Fed. Proc. Fed. Am. Soc. Exp. Biol.,* 39, 884, 1980.
73. **Toth, B., Smith, J., and Patil, K.,** Cancer induction in mice with acetaldehyde methylformylhydrazone of the false morel mushroom, *J. Natl. Cancer Inst.,* 67, 881, 1981.
74. **Toth, B. and Patil, K.,** Gyromitrin as a tumor inducer, *Neoplasma,* 28, 559, 1981.

Chapter 11

FORMATION OF C-NITRO AND C-NITROSO MUTAGENS BY THE REACTION OF NITRITE WITH SORBIC ACID AND ITS ANALOGUES AND THEIR INACTIVATION WITH FOOD CONSTITUENTS

Mitsuo Namiki, Toshihiko Osawa, Tsuneo Kada, Keiichi Tsuji, and Kazuko Namiki

TABLE OF CONTENTS

I. INTRODUCTION

Sorbic acid, or 2,4-hexadienoic acid, is a natural product found in mountain ash berries, and has been used extensively as a safe food preservative with a wide antimicrobial spectrum.* Nitrites have also been used in meat processing as a color fixative and preservative.* The latter is also found naturally in food, especially in vegetables. The relatively early finding that these two common food additives react with each other and produce strong mutagenic activities toward bacteria[1] stimulated us to carry out chemical and biological studies systematically, and a number of the biologically active products of this reaction have been isolated and characterized as various C-nitro and C-nitroso compounds. In contrast to the well investigated studies on mutagen formation by the reaction of nitrite with secondary amines, those by the action of nitrite on unsaturated C-C systems have received only limited attention.[2] Continued studies on the natural analogues of sorbic acid as a suspected mutagen source as well as on the inhibitory effects of commonly present food constituents have been done; the summarized results are reviewed and discussed here.

II. MUTAGEN FORMATION BY THE REACTION OF NITRITE WITH SORBIC ACID

In a very early work,* equimolar amounts of sorbic acid and sodium nitrite were simply mixed under no pH control,[3] but it was shown later that the reaction pH greatly influenced development of the mutagenicity as well as the growth inhibitory activity.[4] Results of the bioassays obtained by the pH controlled reaction are shown in Table 1. The reaction mixture prepared at pH above 6.0 was inactive both in the rec-assay and in the growth inhibition assay. Below this pH, the DNA damaging activity was produced at pHs between 2 to 5, with the maximum at 3.5 to 4.2. The growth inhibitory activity was intensified by lowering the pH to 1.5.

The effect of the reaction pH on the produced mutagenicity was successfully correlated to the results of the chemical composition of the reaction mixtures. All but the main products isolated from the ethyl acetate extract of the reaction mixture have been identified as shown in Figure 1 and, among these, ethylnitrolic acid (ENA) is the only known compound. The biological activities of the reaction mixtures are considered to depend on the distributions of these products. HPLC study of the reaction mixtures prepared under the controlled pH[5] showed that a product named Y̲ is produced by the reaction at pHs between 2.5 and 5.0 with a maximum at 3.0, and ENA, between pH 3.0 and 5.0 with a maximum at 4.2 (Figure 2A). At pH 1.5 the main products were one named B̲ and other minor ones. These are in good accord with the specific activities of the individual products shown in Figure 1 and with the aforementioned pH effect on the produced activities.

Differential product distributions may be caused by dissociation phenomena of the reactants and the complex equilibria among reactive nitrogen oxide species. As shown in Figure 2B, a molar ratio (8:1) of nitrite to sorbic acid optimum for the mutagenicity production was employed in the above studies, but this ratio will not occur in our actual food consumption habit. However, the mutagenicity was detected by the rec-assay method even in the 1:1 reaction mixture. The formation of mutagenic products at this ratio was also confirmed by HPLC analyses. This seems noteworthy considering the safety problem, and is also interesting from a chemical viewpoint because the formation of the product Y̲ seems to require a 4:1 molar ratio.

---

*   Regulated levels in foods: (1) Sorbic acid, below 2 g/kg in fish meat sausage, meat products, etc. (in Japan). 0.05 to 0.02% in chocolate syrup, 0.05 to 0.1% in cheesecake, etc. (in U.S.). 0.2% is approximately 2 × 10^{-2} *M*. (2) Residual nitrite, 0.07 g/kg in meat products and fish meat sausage (in Japan) and 120 ppm in bacon (in U.S.).

Table 1
**pH AND MOLAR EFFECTS ON GENERATION OF DNA-DAMAGING
AND GROWTH-INHIBITORY ACTIVITIES BY REACTION BETWEEN
SORBIC ACID (SA) AND SODIUM NITRITE (SN)[a]**

pH	Dose (μℓ/disk)	Rec-assay, mm of inhibition[b]			Growth inhibition (effective dilution)
		Rec+	Rec−	Activity[c]	
1.5	20	0.5	0	−	+ + + (×3000)
3.0	20	0	1.8	+	+ + (×2000)
3.5	20	1.0	7.4	+ +	+ + (×2000)
4.2	20	2.0	11.7	+ +	+ + (×2000)
5.0	20	0	2.5	+	+ (×400)
6.0	20	0	0	−	− (×200)
7.0	20	0	0	−	− (×200)
Positive control	Mitomycin (0.2 μg)	0	15.0	+ + +	

Molar ratio for reaction (mM)		μℓ per disk	Rec-assay with *B. subtilis*	
			Inhibition (mm)	
SA	SN		Rec+	Rec−
20	0.4	100	0	0
20	2.0	100	0	0
20	20.0	100	0	1.1
20	80.0	50	0	4.6
20	160.0	20	2.9	10.8
20	320.0	20	3.0	9.0

[a]   Sorbic acid (20 mM) and sodium nitrite (160 mM) were reacted at 60°C for 1 hr.
[b]   Cold incubation method.
[c]   Based on the difference of inhibition zones: −, less than 1 mm; +, 1 to 5 mm; + +, more than 5 mm.

From Namiki, M., *J. Agric. Food Chem.*, 29, 407, 1981. With permission.

III. MUTAGEN FORMATION BY THE REACTION OF NITRITE WITH SORBIC ACID ANALOGOUS FOOD CONSTITUENTS[8]

Sorbic acid is a simple dienoic carboxylic acid, however, there are many food components and additives having the partial structures analogous to sorbic acid. Therefore, it seems very important from the viewpoint of food safety to elucidate the potential of these compounds in mutagen production by the reaction with nitrite. These studies will also help in understanding the general reaction mechanisms and the structure-activity relationships of mutagens of this type.

The compounds examined among food constituents that are analogous to sorbic acid and their mutagenicities produced by the reaction with nitrite are shown in Figure 3. The compounds having no dienoic carbonyl, i.e., crotonic acid, crotonaldehyde, oleic acid, and furfural did not provide any detectable reaction products on TLC and showed no induction of mutagenicity. On the other hand, sorbic acid methyl ester and piperine gave several detectable reaction products on TLC and exhibited strong mutagenicities. 2-Furanacrylic acid, β-carotene, and tung oil, having conjugated diene or polyene, gave significant amounts of the reaction products including weak mutagens. These results may suggest that the conjugated dienoic carbonyl group is essential for mutagen formation by the reactions with nitrite.

	Products		Mutagenicity			Growth inhibition
			Rec-assay	Ames-assay		
				TA-98	TA-100	
	Ethylnitrolic acid (ENA)	$O_2N\!-\!C(\!=\!NOH)\!-\!CH_3$	++	−	+	+
	1,4-dinitro-2-methyl pyrrol (product Y)	(pyrrole structure)	+++	++	++	+
	Product-B	(structure) or (structure)	−	−	−	+++
	Product-F	(structure)	−	−	−	−
	Precursor-F (syn- + anti-)	(structure)	−	−	−	−

Sorbic acid (SA)

+

$NaNO_2$

Sodium Nitrite (SN)

FIGURE 1. Biological activities of individual isolated products and reactants. For details of the bioassay see Reference 4.

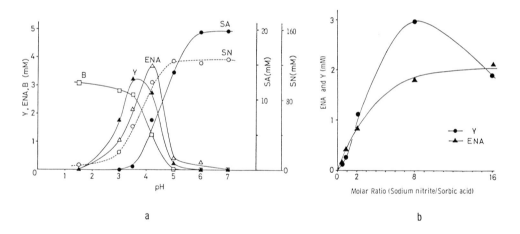

FIGURE 2. Effects of reaction pH and molar ratio on the formation of the reaction products of sorbic acid with sodium nitrite. Sorbic acid (20 mM) with sodium nitrite (160 mM) were reacted at 60°C for 30 min. Reaction products were quantified by HPLC. (μ-Bondapak C_{18}. Solvent: H_2O-methanol 85:15).

Isolation and identification of the reaction products by means of TLC, HPLC, and various instrumental analyses indicated that the main mutagen formed by the nitrite-sorbic acid methyl ester reaction is 5-nitro-2,4-hexadienoic acid methyl ester.[8] ENA was also isolated from this reaction mixture, although its formation was relatively slow and low in yield as compared with those in the case of sorbic acid. The difference between the methyl ester and free sorbic acid in the products is still not fully explained.

The positive result with the piperine-nitrite system poses a serious safety problem because the piperine content of pepper is as high as 5% and pepper is very widely used in cooking and meat processing, frequently in the presence of nitrite. The mutagenicity produced in the piperine-nitrite system was far stronger than that in the sorbic acid-nitrite system.[9]

Material Compound	Structure	Product	Mutagenicity	
			Rec-assay	Ames-assay (TA 98)
Sorbic acid	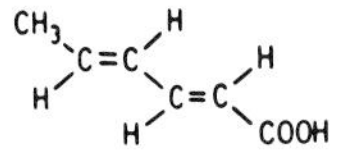 [structure]	E N A Y B F Pre-F	+ ++ - - -	- ++ - - -
Sorbic acid methyl ester	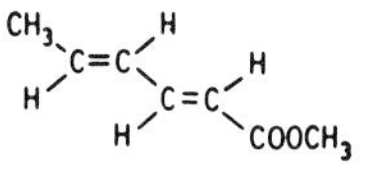 [structure]	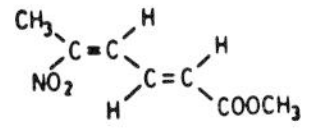 E N A [structure] 5-Nitro-2,4-hexadienoic acid methyl ester	+ ++	- -
Crotonic acid	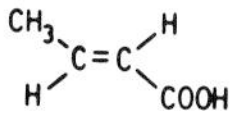 [structure]	N D	-	NT
Crotonaldehyde	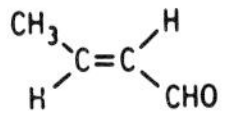 [structure]	N D	-	NT
Furfural	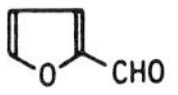 [structure]	N D	-	NT
2-Furanacrylic acid	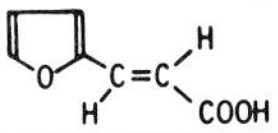 [structure]	unknown	+	NT
Oleic acid	$CH_3(CH_2)_7CH=CH(CH_2)_7COOH$	N D	-	NT
β-Carotene	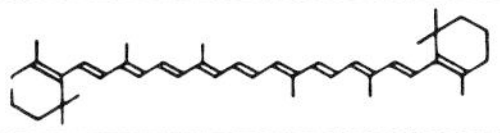 [structure]	unknown	±	NT
Piperine	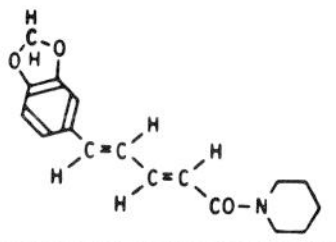 [structure]	unknown	++	+++
Tung oil	trans trans cis $CH_3(CH_2)_3CH \cdot CHCH \cdot CHCH \cdot CH(CH_2)_7COOH$ α-Eleostearic acid (Main component of tung oil)	N D	-	NT

N D ; not detected   NT ; not tested

FIGURE 3. Mutagen formation by the reaction of sorbic acid analogues with sodium nitrite. For details of the bioassay see Reference 8.

Investigations on the nitrite-piperine reaction mixture by means of TLC along with the mutagenicity tests (Figure 4A) indicated that two main fractions, Numbers 2 and 7 were active without metabolic activation in the strains TA100 and TA98; the fraction Number 1 was very active especially in TA100. Formation of *N*-nitroso piperidine, a well known mutagen, by the reaction of nitrite with piperine in acid solution has already been reported,[10] but its contribution to the mutagenicities of the above mentioned TLC fractions was excluded by the following facts: (1) the Rf value of an authentic *N*-nitrosopiperidine on TLC under the same condition (0.52) was apparently different from that of the detected mutagen, (2) mutagenicity of *N*-nitrosopiperidine was known to be observed only in the presence of S9 mix in the Ames test,[11] and (3) the mutagenic fractions Numbers 1, 2, and 7 could be detected on TLC of the reaction mixture of nitrite-piperic acid system.

Thus it is evident that the mutagenic products from piperine or piperic acid are apparently different from *N*-nitrosopiperidine, and are the products of the action of nitrite on the dienoic moiety of piperine or piperic acid.

By a preparative scale reaction of piperic acid and sodium nitrite at pH 3.5, one of the main mutagenic products was obtained as crystalline form, and identified as 6-nitro-piperonal by chemical analyses. Formation reaction is assumed as shown in Figure 4B. One of the other mutagenic products having a potent activity was isolated, but it was unstable and not yet obtained as a pure product.

IV. EFFECTS OF FOOD CONSTITUENTS ON C-NITRO AND C-NITROSO MUTAGEN FORMATION AND THE MUTAGENICITY OF THE REACTION PRODUCTS

A. Inhibition of Mutagen Formation

Inhibitory effects of ascorbic acid and cysteine have been shown on the formation of *N*-nitrosamine, mainly due to the competitive action of ascorbic acid to amine with nitrite. A similar effect of ascorbic acid or cysteine was observed on C-nitro mutagen formation by the nitrite-sorbic acid reaction, that is, addition of a half molar equivalent of ascorbic acid or an equivalent molar of cysteine nearly eliminate the mutagen formation.[5]

B. Desmutagenic Actions of Food Components on C-Nitro Mutagens

The vegetables which were effective in eliminating the mutagenicity of the nitrite-sorbic acid system are listed in Table 2. The homogenates prepared from pumpkin, field pea, yam, green peas, and ginkgo nuts showed marked desmutagenic activities. It was also demonstrated by HPLC analysis that the treatment of Y with pumpkin juice brought about a marked decrease of Y at pH 6.8, though it was slight at pH 5.0. (Figure 5). Because Y is a main mutagen formed by the nirite-sorbic reaction, the desmutagenic action of the vegetable juices on the mutagenicity generated in that system might be greatly due to degradation of Y with the vegetable juice.

Further investigations on various food constituents showed that several substances having a reducing power such as ascorbic acid and cysteine are effective in the desmutagenic activity on Y. As shown in Figure 5, the desmutagenic action of ascorbic acid and cysteine was effective only at neutral pH, which was supported by the HPLC data indicating a marked degradation of Y by a similar treatment. These results suggest that ascorbic acid, cysteine, and other reducing substances might greatly contribute to the desmutagenic action of pumpkin and other vegetable juices. HPLC analysis of the reaction mixture indicated that Y was altered mostly to a new product, which was identified as the reduced product of C-nitro to C-amino group of Y by NMR and MS analyses, and which has no biological activity.

Inactivation of the mutagenicity of 6-nitropiperonal formed by the reaction of nitrite with piperine was also observed by the treatment of ascorbic acid, cysteine, and other reducing substances. The effect of ascorbic acid was also assumed to be caused by the reduction of the conjugated C-nitro group, while that of cysteine seemed different and the inactivation mechanism may involve direct attack of cysteine to the aromatic ring of Y or 6-nitropiperonal along with subsequent elimination of the C-nitro group as well as its mutagenicity.

V. SUMMARY

The development of mutagenicity by the reaction of nitrite with sorbic acid is highly dependent upon the reaction conditions, especially pH, being maximum at pH 3.5 but negative at pH 6.0 or above. We succeeded in the isolation and identification of the main reaction products and found that most mutagens are new C-nitro and C-nitroso compounds. Investigations on the reactions of nitrite with various food constituents led to the assumption that the conjugated dienoic carbonyl structure is essential for mutagen formation, though details of the formation mechanism of the C-nitro and nitroso products still remain obscure.

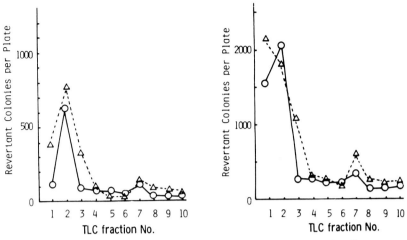

Mutagenicity of TLC Fractions of Products of Pierine-Nitrite Reaction

—O— : Piperine(0.1 mM) + NaNO$_2$(0.8 mM) (−S-9 mix)

--△-- : Piperic acid(0.1 mM) + NaNO$_2$(0.8 mM) (−S-9 mix)

TLC: Wako Gel FM plate, n-hexane:acetic acid: ethyl acetate:Chloroform(45:6:10:1)

Formation of C-Nitro Mutagens by Piperine-Nitrite Reaction

FIGURE 4. Mutagenicity of TLC fractions of products and proposed formation pathway of C-nitro mutagens by the piperine-nitrite reaction. The ethyl acetate extract from 4 mℓ of each reaction mixture was separated by a preparative TLC. After development of the plate, 10 equal zones were fractionated and the mutagenicity of each fraction was determined in the Ames test using *Salmonella typhimurium* TA100 and 98 without S9 mix.

Among the food constituents, the nitrite-piperine or piperic acid reaction was found to give strong mutagens and one of them was identified as 6-nitropiperonal. We also demonstrated that many kinds of common vegetable juices as well as ascorbic acid and cysteine inactivate effectively mutagenicities of the C-nitro mutagens, especially those of Y and 6-nitropiperonal. Fortunately, compared to *N*-nitroso mutagens, the C-nitro mutagens formed by the reaction of nitrite with food constituents are shown to be more susceptible to the inactivating action of various food constituents, especially such reducing substances as ascorbic acid and cysteine. Further studies on the development of these new types of mutagens in the course of practical food processing as well as in the digestion are being undertaken.

Table 2
DESMUTAGENIC FOOD ACTING ON MUTAGENIC PRODUCTS GENERATED BY SORBIC ACID WITH SODIUM NITRITE

Remarkable	Moderate	
Pumpkin	Spinach	Japanese pear
Field pea	Cabbage	Pear
Yam	Lettuce	Japanese pepper
Green peas	Green pepper	Carrot
Ginkgo nut	Tomato	Enokidake mushroom
	Mint	Shimeji mushroom
	Honewort	Bofu
	Red cabbage	Dropwort
	Chinese cabbage	Rape blossoms
	Eggplant	Mint (leaf)
	Asparagus	Beet
	Cauliflower	Snowpea
	Beetsteak plant	Broccoli
	Indian lotus	Artichoke
	Mandarin orange	Alfalfa sprout
	Banana	Yellow squash
	Pineapple	Oats
		Long yam

Note: After the reaction of sorbic acid with sodium nitrite at pH 3.5 and room temperature for 24 hr, a portion of the reaction mixture was mixed with the preparation of each food homogenate and assayed by the rec-assay. If a food sample abolished the positive rec-assay effect of mutagenic products, we conclude its desmutagenicity.

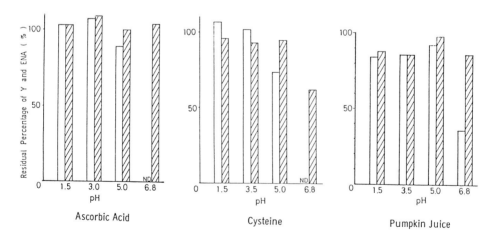

FIGURE 5.   Degradation of 1,4-dinitro-2-methyl pyrrole (Y) and ethylnitrolic acid (ENA) by treatment with ascorbic acid, cysteine, or pumpkin juice (☐ Y; ▨ ENA). Incubation was carried out with or without 8 mM of ascorbic acid or cysteine in 10 mℓ buffer solution of 1 mM Y and ENA. 20 mℓ of pumpkin juice was freeze-dried after filtration and dissolved in 10 mℓ buffer solution of 1 mM Y and ENA. Residual amounts of Y and ENA were quantified by HPLC (μ-Bondapak C$_{18}$. Solvent: H$_2$O-methanol = 85:15).

REFERENCES

1. **Kada, T.,** DNA-damaging products from reaction between sodium nitrite and sorbic acid, *Annu. Rep. Natl. Inst. Genet. (Jpn.)*, 24, 43, 1974.
2. **Pitts, J. N., Jr., Van Cauwenverhge, K. A., Grosjean, D., Schmid, J. P., Fitz, D. R., Belser, W. L., Knudson, G. B., and Hynds, P. M.,** Atmospheric reactions of polycyclic aromatic hydrocarbons: facile formation of mutagenic nitro derivatives, *Science,* 202, 515, 1978.
3. **Namiki, M. and Kada, T.,** Formation of ethylnitrolic acid by the reaction of sorbic acid with sodium nitrite, *Agric. Biol. Chem.,* 39, 1335, 1975.
4. **Namiki, M., Udaka, S., Osawa, T., Tsuji, K., and Kada, T.,** Formation of mutagens by sorbic acid-nitrite reaction: effects of reaction conditions on biological activities, *Mutat. Res.,* 73, 21, 1980.
5. **Namiki, M., Osawa, T., Ishibashi, H., Namiki, K., and Tsuji, K.,** Chemical aspects of mutagen formation by sorbic acid-sodium nitrite reaction, *J. Agric. Food Chem.,* 29, 407, 1981.
6. **Kito, Y. and Namiki, M.,** A new N-nitropyrrole: 1,4-dinitro-2-methylpyrrole, formed by the reaction of sorbic acid with sodium nitrite, *Tetrahedron,* 34, 505, 1978.
7. **Osawa, T., Kito, M., Namiki, M., and Tsuji, K.,** A new furoxan derivative and its precursors formed by the reaction of sorbic acid with sodium nitrite, *Tetrahedron Lett.,* 45, 4399, 1979.
8. **Osawa, T. and Namiki, M.,** Mutagen formation by the reaction of nitrite with the food components analogous to sorbic acid, *Agric. Biol. Chem.,* 46, 2299, 1982.
9. **Lijinsky, W., Conrad, E., and Bogart, R. V.,** Carcinogenic nitrosamines formed by drug/nitrite interaction, *Nature (London),* 239, 165, 1972.
10. **Rao, T. K., Hardigree, A. A., Young, J. A., Lijinsky, W., and Epler, J. L.,** Mutagenicity of N-nitroso-piperidines with *Salmonella typhimurium*/microsomal activation system, *Mutat. Res.,* 56, 131, 1977.
11. **Osawa, T., Ishibashi, H., Namiki, M., Yamanaka, M., and Namiki, K.,** *Mutat. Res.,* 91, 291, 1981.
12. **Osawa, T., Ishibashi, H., Namiki, M., and Kada, T.,** Desmutagenic actions of ascorbic acid and cysteine on a new pyrrole mutagen formed by the reaction between food additives; sorbic acid and sodium nitrite, *Biochem. Biophys. Res. Commun.,* 95, 835, 1980.

Chapter 12

MUTAGEN FORMATION BY THE NITRITE-SPICE REACTION AND ITS INHIBITION

Kazuko Namiki, Toshihiko Osawa, and Mitsuo Namiki

TABLE OF CONTENTS

I. INTRODUCTION

The mutagenicity produced by the chemical reaction between natural or added food constituents is no less important than that of the constituents themselves in food. Beside the well-known example of the formation of *N*-nitrosamines by the reaction of nitrites on secondary amines, that of mutagenic C-nitro and C-nitroso compounds by the reaction of nitrites with sorbic acid, a common food preservative, has been investigated in a series of papers.[1-5]

Continued studies have shown a similar mutagen formation by the reaction of nitrite with several other compounds that have a common partial structure of conjugated dienoic carbonyl.[6] Because piperine, a main pungent principle of pepper, showed a very strong mutagenic activity by the reaction with nitrite, the study was extended to the investigation of the reaction of pepper powder[7] and other common commercial spices with nitrite.

By the standard Ames test using *Salmonella typhimurium* TA98 and TA100, nitrite-treated pepper, nutmeg, laurel, chili pepper, and others were found to be significantly mutagenic. The effect of reaction pH, temperature, and nitrite concentration on the produced mutagenicity was examined. Pepper powder was found to produce detectable amounts of mutagens by reaction with nitrite at lower concentration, which is the legally permitted level in meat and other food products; this seemed important from the viewpoint of practical food safety.

The extracts of the various mutagenic reaction mixtures were fractionated by preparative TLC, and the mutagenicity from these spices was located in at least four different fractions. One of them was identical with the purified product of the reaction of piperine, but the other two were different products.

The stability of the unfractionated reaction products from pepper toward heat was examined. Also, the possible effect of common food constituents and raw vegetable juices on the reaction of nitrite with spices, and desmutagenic activities were examined.[8]

The results of these past studies are reviewed and discussed in the following sections.

II. COMPARISON OF SPICES

The results of the Ames test on the products of the reaction of nitrite with 14 different commercially available spice powders are shown in Figure 1. The figures show strong mutagenicity for pepper, nutmeg, laurel, chili pepper, wuxiangfen, and others. The blank tests using the solvent extracts of the untreated spices showed negative mutagenicity in all cases.

III. EFFECT OF REACTION CONDITIONS

The effect of the reaction pH on the produced mutagenicity was studied according to the method described in the former section. As shown in Figure 2, the mutagenicity produced from pepper and nutmeg both becomes maximum at pH 3.0 to 3.5.

Higher reaction temperature enhanced the production of mutagenicity, and virtually no mutagenicity was detected after 3 hr of the reaction at 5°C (Figure 3).

The lower limit of the nitrite concentration for mutagen formation was examined in relation to the normal conditions of food consumption. The maximum legally permitted level of nitrite in animal or fish meat is usually between 50 to 100 mg/kg. In addition, the amount of nitrite derived from the nitrate in vegetables can sometimes be considerable. The amount of spices consumed for a dish of cooked meat would usually be between 0.2 and 0.5 g. Taking these into consideration, an experiment at the lower nitrite levels was carried out and the results are shown in Figure 4. It was shown that the mutagenicity produced was significant even at these lower levels, and was stronger with pepper than with nutmeg.

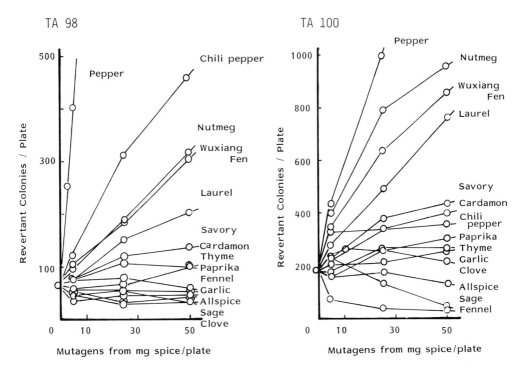

FIGURE 1. Mutagenicity produced by spice-nitrite reaction. Spice powder (5 g) and NaNO₂ (0.55 g) were mixed in 200 mℓ of the medium (pH 3.5 McIlvaine buffer, 20% EtOH) and the resultant suspension was warmed at 40°C for 20 hr, filtered, and extracted 3 times with ethyl acetate. The concentrated extract was dissolved in EtOH for the Ames test. Ames test was carried out with *Salmonella typhimurium* TA98 and TA100, without metabolic activation. Equivalent weights of spices per plate in the Ames test are shown.

IV. MUTAGENICITY OF FRACTIONATED REACTION MIXTURES

The reaction mixtures of pepper and nutmeg were extracted as described and fractionated on silica gel (Wakogel®) TLC plates (Figure 5) with a solvent system hexane-acetic acid-ethyl acetate-chloroform (90:9:12:2). The mutagenic activities from the reaction mixture of pepper appeared in fractions 2 and 7 among the 10 numbered fractions. On the other hand, the main mutagenicity of the nutmeg-nitrite, laurel-nitrite, and other reaction mixture was located at fraction 1 and was apparently of a different identity from the mutagenic fractions formed by the pepper-nitrite reaction.

V. THE EFFECT OF S9 MIX ON MUTAGENICITY

The effect of metabolic activation of the mutagenic products was investigated using the S9 mix (0.3 mℓ per plate) prepared from rat liver homogenate induced by phenobarbital. The Ames test with TA98 strain showed a significant suppression of the activities of the pepper-nitrite and nutmeg-nitrite reaction mixtures and, with the TA100 strain, the effect was dependent on the dose of the reaction mixtures. Some enhancement was observed at higher doses (Figure 6).

VI. HEAT STABILITY OF THE MUTAGENICITY

When the mutagenic reaction mixture (124 mg pepper or nutmeg + 12 mg NaNO₂ in 100 mℓ pH 3.5 buffer, 20 hr at 40°C) was adjusted for pH and kept at boiling bath temperature for 2 hr, about 30% of the activity before heating was lost at pH 6.5. The loss was minimal at pH 3.5.

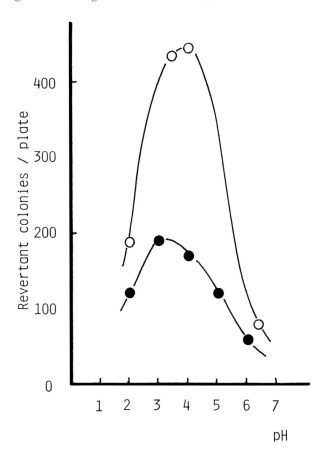

FIGURE 2.   Effect of reaction pH on the produced mutagenicity. Reaction procedure same as Figure 1 except for pH. Ames test was carried out with *Salmonella typhimurium* TA98, without metabolic activation (-○- pepper-nitrite, -●- nutmeg-nitrite).

VII. EFFECT OF COMMON FOOD CONSTITUENTS ON MUTAGEN FORMATION AND MUTAGENICITY OF THE REACTION PRODUCTS

The effect of the presence of other constituents of food on the mutagen-forming reaction and on the already formed mutagenic products may not be disregarded under normal conditions of food consumption. The pepper-nitrite mixture was reacted in the presence of various conceivable food constituents. The presence of sugars apparently had no effect on the produced mutagenicity. Among amino acids, cysteine and tryptophan significantly suppressed the mutagen formation, though methionine was less effective. On the other hand, α-alanine or its mixture with glucose as additives rather enhanced the activity. Vitamins, retinol, ascorbic acid, and α-tocopherol also showed suppressive effects. Raw vegetable juices generally suppressed the mutagen formation, and juice containing vegetable pulp seemed more effective in general (Figure 7).

Desmutagenic actions of food constituents were also investigated by adding the food constituents to the reaction mixture of pepper with nitrite for 20 hr at room temperature at pH 3.5 or 6.5, and assayed by the Ames test (Figure 8). The desmutagenic effect seemed more marked by the treatment at pH 6.5. Ascorbic acid, α-tocopherol, cysteine, and tryptophan reduced the activity to 40 to 50%, and vegetable juice, to less than 30%, when the tester strain was TA98. The effect was less marked with the TA100 strain.

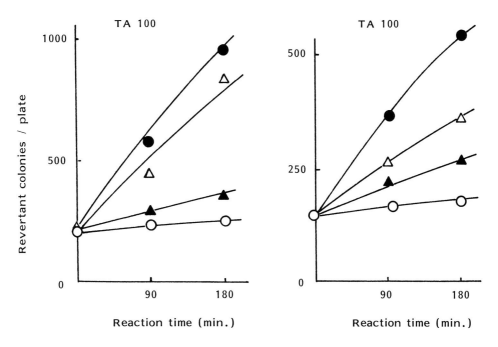

FIGURE 3. Effect of temperature on the produced mutagenicity. Reaction procedure same as in Figure 1 except for temperature. (Left) Pepper powder; (right) nutmeg powder. Equivalent milligrams of the spices are shown. Ames test was carried out without metabolic activation (-●- 60°C, -△- 40°C, -▲- 20°C, -○- 5°C).

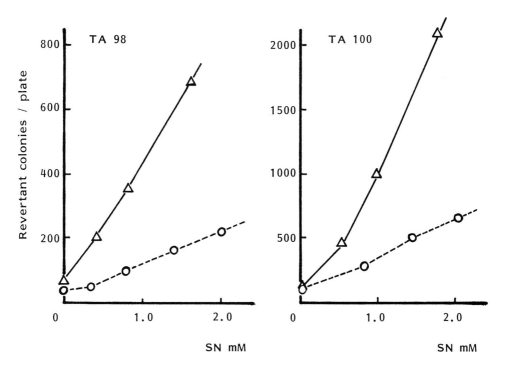

FIGURE 4. Effect of nitrite concentration in the reaction on the mutagenicity. The amount of the spice was 1 g/1000 mℓ and sodium nitrite concentration was 0.4 to 2.0 mM. The reaction was continued for 20 hr at 40°C at pH 3.5 (-△- pepper-nitrite, -○- nutmeg-nitrite).

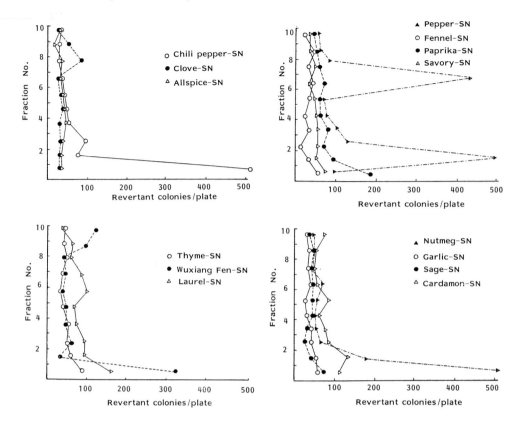

FIGURE 5. Fractionation of the reaction mixtures on TLC plate. The concentrated extract of the reaction mixture obtained by the procedure of Figure 1 was developed on silica gel plate (Wakogel®) using a solvent system n-hexane-acetic acid-ethyl acetate-chloroform (90:9:12:2). The fractions scraped off the plates were assayed by the Ames method.

VIII. CONCLUSION

The results summarized indicate that the possibility of mutagen formation by the reaction of certain kinds of common spices with nitrites cannot be disregarded. Pepper and nutmeg produced particularly potent mutagens of different identities. Pepper at least was capable of producing significant mutagenicity under normal conditions of food consumption.

The mutagen formation and mutagenicity seem to be counteracted by the addition of common food constituents. The mutagenicity showed a tendency to be weakened by the presence of S9 mix. The meaning of these findings from the viewpoint of food safety should be clarified by further studies under conditions closer to real-life food consumption.

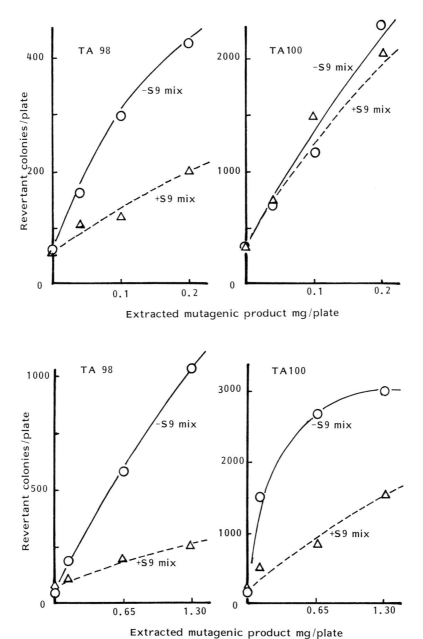

FIGURE 6. Effect of metabolic activation by S9 mix. S9 mix (0.3 mℓ) was used in this experiment. S9 mix was purchased from the Oriental Yeast Company. (Top) Pepper-nitrite (TA98, TA100); (bottom) nutmeg-nitrite (TA98, TA100).

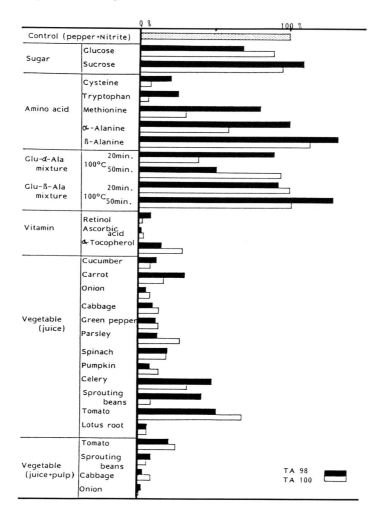

FIGURE 7.   Effect of addition of common food constituents and vegetable juices on mutagen formation by pepper-nitrite reaction. White pepper (124 mg) + NaNO$_2$(12 mg) was reacted for 20 hr at 40°C, in 100 mℓ of the medium (pH 3.5 McIlvaine buffer, 20% EtOH) in the presence of 0.17 mmol of the pure additive or one of the vegetable juices equivalent to 40 g each of fresh materials.

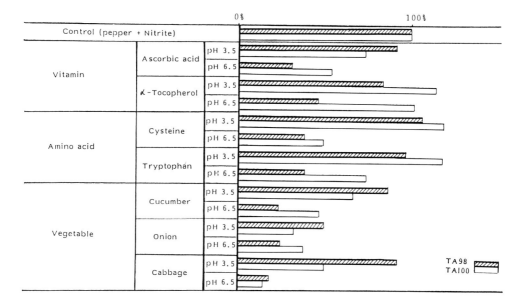

FIGURE 8. Effect of food constituents on the mutagenicity of the pepper-nitrite reaction product. Pepper-nitrite mixture (as in Figure 7) after the reaction was mixed with 0.17 mmol of the pure additive or one of the vegetable juices equivalent to 40 g of fresh materials and kept for 20 hr at room temperature. The extracts of these mixtures were used for the Ames test.

REFERENCES

1. **Kada, T.**, DNA-damaging products from reaction between sodium nitrite and sorbic acid, *Annu. Rep. Natl. Inst. Genet. (Jpn.)*, 24, 43, 1974.
2. **Namiki, M. and Kada, T.**, Formation of ethylnitrolic acid by the reaction of sorbic acid with sodium nitrite, *Agric. Biol. Chem.*, 39, 1335, 1975.
3. **Namiki, M., Udaka, S., Osawa, T., Tsuji, K., and Kada, T.**, Formation of mutagens by sorbic acid-nitrite reaction: effects of reaction conditions on biological activities, *Mutat. Res.*, 73, 21, 1980.
4. **Namiki, M., Osawa, T., Ishibashi, H., Namiki, K., and Tsuji, K.**, Chemical aspects of mutagen formation by sorbic acid-sodium nitrite reaction, *J. Agric. Food Chem.*, 29, 407, 1981.
5. **Osawa, T., Kito, M., Namiki, M., and Tsuji, K.**, A new furoxan derivative and its precursors formed by the reaction of sorbic acid with sodium nitrite, *Tetrahedron Lett.*, 45, 4399, 1979.
6. **Osawa, T., Namiki, M., and Namiki, K.**, Mutagen formation in the nitrite-piperic acid reaction, *Agric. Biol. Chem.*, 46, 12, 1982.
7. **Osawa, T., Ishibashi, H., Namiki, M., Yamanaka, M., and Namiki, K.**, Formation of mutagens by pepper-nitrite reaction, *Mutat. Res.*, 91, 291, 1981.
8. **Osawa, T., Ishibashi, H., Namiki, M., and Kada, T.**, Desmutagenic actions of ascorbic acid and cysteine on a new pyrrole mutagen formed by the reaction between food additives; sorbic acid and sodium nitrite, *Biochem. Biophys. Res. Commun.*, 95, 835, 1980.

Chapter 13

CARCINOGENIC AND MUTAGENIC MYCOTOXINS

D. R. Stoltz

TABLE OF CONTENTS

I. INTRODUCTION

Doll and Peto[1] have recently estimated that dietary factors account for 35% of cancer deaths in the U.S. Tobacco, with an estimated contribution of 30% of all cancer deaths, was followed distantly by infections (10%), reproductive and sexual behavior (7%), and occupation, alcohol, geophysical factors, food additives, pollution, industrial products, and medicines, each causing less than 5% of the cancer deaths.

Five possible ways or means whereby diet may affect the incidence of cancer were suggested: (1) ingestion of powerful, direct-acting carcinogens or their precursors; (2) altering the formation of carcinogens in the body; (3) influencing transport, activation, or deactivation of carcinogens; (4) affecting promotion of cells that are already initiated; and (5) overnutrition. In the context of current theories of carcinogenesis the first three mechanisms relate to initiation, either obviously, such as ingestion of the initiator, aflatoxin, or of nitrite, a precursor of initiating N-nitroso-compounds, or indirectly through deactivation of initiators by vitamin E. Other dietary constituents or lack of them may affect cancer incidence by acting after initiation at the promotion stage (e.g., croton oil, vitamin A deficiency) or at later stages in tumor progression.

Where there appears to be consensus that the natural course of neoplastic development may be divided into at least three different stages, namely initiation, promotion, and progression,[2,3] there is less agreement upon the terms presently applied to agents or conditions which affect the different stages.[4,5] In the present discussion it is assumed that mutation is the critical event in initiation and that mutagenic chemicals are potential initiators of carcinogenesis. Furthermore, promoters, enhancing agents, positive modifiers, or incomplete carcinogens are agents that induce tumors in an intact mammal and enhance the carcinogenicity of initiators, but are not mutagenic. Complete carcinogens possess both initiating and promoting activities. Although reliance upon ''mutation'' in these definitions may prove to be too restrictive, alternative terms such as ''genotoxicity'' presently lack precision.

The possibility that mycotoxins might contribute to neoplastic development by any means other than as initiators has received little attention. Immunosuppression by *Fusarium* products and estrogenic action of zearalenone are potential examples that might warrant investigation.[6] Furthermore, the very real possibility that fungal toxins other than aflatoxin might contribute to the large proportion of cancer deaths attributed to dietary factors accentuates the need to search for such toxins and to investigate their modes of action with modern toxicity screens. This discussion concerns fungal products that might contaminate food rather than toxins which are constituents of edible mushrooms.

II. CARCINOGENIC MYCOTOXINS

Several recent authoritative reviews[6-9] convey the impression that a number of fungal metabolites are carcinogenic but in some cases the experimental evidence is not compelling. A tabulation of mycotoxins with confirmed carcinogenic activity for experimental animals lists seven compounds (Table 1) chosen on the basis of the strength of evidence for carcinogenicity. A further ten toxins (Table 2) have demonstrated insufficient evidence of carcinogenicity in limited or contradictory animal studies.

The confirmed animal carcinogens (Table 1) which are mutagenic in bacterial short-term predictive tests should be considered initiators or complete carcinogens. The exceptions, luteoskyrin[10] and griseofulvin[8] are apparently not mutagenic, but require further investigation. The mycotoxins with insufficient evidence of carcinogenic activity (Table 2) are generally not mutagenic for bacteria, although isolated positive responses in some ''genotoxicity tests'' have been reported. This lack of bacterial mutagenicity, coupled with difficulty in eliciting carcinogenicity in traditional bioassays, suggests that if these toxins have any effect at all upon neoplastic development, it is at some stage after initiation or in some role other than as initiator.

Table 1
MYCOTOXINS: CONFIRMED
CARCINOGENS[8,17]

Mycotoxin	Target tissue
Aflatoxin B_1,G_1,M_1	Liver, kidney
Coumarin	Liver
Griseofulvin	Liver
Luteoskyrin	Liver
Sterigmatocystin	Liver, lung, skin

Table 2
MYCOTOXINS: SELECTED EXAMPLES OF COMPOUNDS WITH
EQUIVOCAL EVIDENCE OF CARCINOGENICITY

Mycotoxin	Comments
Citrinin	Kidney tumor enhancer, unconfirmed[32]
Cyclochlorotine	Hepatocarcinogen, unconfirmed[57]
Ochratoxin A	Liver and kidney carcinogen, unconfirmed[31]
Patulin	Injection site sarcomas only[24]
Penicillic acid	Injection site sarcomas only[24]
Psoralens	Photocarcinogenic; phytoalexin rather than mycotoxin?[11,13]
Rugulosin	Hepatocarcinogen, unconfirmed[47]
T-2 toxin, trichothecenes	Esophageal carcinogen or promoter?[28,30,33,58]
Zearalenone	Mammary, pituitary, and hepatocellular adenomas, unconfirmed[59,60]

Table 3
MYCOTOXINS MUTAGENIC FOR
SALMONELLA: NO INFORMATION ON
CARCINOGENICITY

Alternariol methylether[52]	Kojic acid[10,63]
Austdiol[10]	Lumiluteoskyrin[64]
Austocystins[10]	Mollicellins[65]
Botryodiplodin[61]	Physcion[51]
Chrysophanol[62]	Physcionanthrones[51]
Emodin[62]	Rubroskyrin[64]
Erythroglaucin[51]	Simatoxin[64]
Fusarin C[53]	Viridicatumtoxin[10]

The broad application of bacterial mutagenicity assays for screening potentially carcinogenic agents has resulted in a growing list of mutagenic fungal products for which no animal cancer bioassay data presently exist (Table 3). These compounds must be considered good candidates for initiators and tested in appropriate animal bioassays.

Psoralens, arbitrarily placed in Table 2, may be used to illustrate more than one problem in mycotoxicology. To begin, since psoralens occur naturally in some plants and accumulate in response to stress, there remains controversy as to whether they are indeed fungal products.[11,12] Nevertheless, it is clear that PUVA (psoralen photochemotherapy, 8-methoxypsoralen + UV-A) is carcinogenic for mouse skin.[13] Although psoralens are both photomutagenic and apparently directly mutagenic in the dark, the effect of metabolism upon mutagenicity remains to be clarified.[14] Experiments to distinguish which of 8-methoxypsoralen, its metabolites of UV-A irradiation, either singly or in combination, acts to initiate and/or promote mouse skin cancer have not been reported.[15]

Although coumarin (Table 1) is not generally appreciated as a fungal product, it has been identified as an in vitro metabolite of *Phytophthora infestans*.[16] Since coumarin has commercial potential as a flavor and odor enhancing agent, reports of carcinogenicity have been rigorously scrutinized and disputed. While marked species and strain differences in metabolism may contribute to divergent results in animal bioassays,[17] two reports indicate mutagenic activity for *Salmonella*.[18,19]

Of the compounds presently with solid evidence of carcinogenicity, only aflatoxins and sterigmatocystin have been reported to occur in the food supply as a result of fungal contamination. The considerable potential for exposure to those toxins with marginal evidence of carcinogenicity, such as *Fusarium* metabolites, ochratoxins, and patulin, has been well documented. In many instances, the environmental distribution of those toxins with mutagenicity but no carcinogenicity data is not known.[20]

Tables 2 and 3 contain selected examples of mycotoxins in the respective categories. Closely related compounds and precursors, especially of aflatoxins, are not catalogued here. For these details and for information regarding nonmutagenic toxins and results of other "genotoxicity" tests, the reader is referred to several recent reviews.[6-9]

III. SCREENING MYCOTOXINS FOR CARCINOGENICITY

Carcinogenicity assessment of recognized mycotoxins should proceed within the framework of currently postulated mechanisms of carcinogenesis. Thus, bacterial mutation assays predict initiating activity with reasonable confidence and low cost, while a broader range of steps in carcinogenesis may be encompassed with an in vitro cell transformation assay.[21] Limited in vivo cancer bioassays[22] capable of responding to initiators and promoters should be applied to all fungal metabolites showing evidence of activity in these short-term tests and/or for which potential human exposure is thought to be significant.

Concern has been voiced over the production of false negatives in the *Salmonella* assay and the requirement of additional microbial tests, particularly the rec-assay and yeast systems to supplement *Salmonella* for detection of genetic activity of mycotoxins.[8,9] Patulin and penicillic acid were cited as examples. Although both patulin and penicillic acid have been tested by several routes of administration, tumors have only been produced by repeated s.c. injection, and then only local tumors were observed.[23,24] Thus, these two mycotoxins provide examples of false positive responses to the s.c. injection method rather than false negatives in the *Salmonella* mutagenicity test. Despite the foregoing, false negative results might be anticipated for both "metabolic" and "mechanistic" reasons. In the former instance, a false negative result could be due to failure of the tissue homogenate to approximate mammalian metabolism. "Mechanistic" false negatives in the *Salmonella* assay can result if the carcinogen acts by some mechanism other than mutation or by a mutation not detected by the *Salmonella* strains.

The mutagenic toxins for which there is no information on carcinogenicity (Table 3) should be given high priority for testing in in vivo assays of initiating activity such as mouse skin[25] and rat liver foci[26] assays. A number of chemicals and complex mixtures have been examined in the mouse skin assay by topical and systemic administration routes of the suspected initiator followed by promotion with croton oil or purified phorbol esters. The rat liver foci bioassay, reviewed recently by Pereira,[26] has rapidly accumulated proponents during its relatively short history of use. Unfortunately, few mycotoxins have been tested in these assays: aflatoxin B_1 was positive in the rat liver foci[27] and mouse skin assays, when assayed for initiating activity,[28] while coumarin[29] and T-2 toxin[30] were negative as initiators in the mouse skin painting assay.

Compounds with insufficient or contradictory evidence of carcinogenicity (Table 2) are prime candidates for promoters and should be assessed for such activity in the mouse skin[25] and rat liver foci[26] assays. Again, only a few mycotoxins have been specifically examined for tumor promoting activity and then only in the mouse skin assay: T-2 toxin[28,30] and diacetoxyscirpenol[28] showed equivocal promoting activity on 7,12-dimethyl-benz(a)anthracene (DMBA)-initiated skin but no activity when aflatoxin B_1 was employed as initiator. Aflatoxin failed to promote DMBA-initiated skin.[28] A report that ochratoxin A enhanced aflatoxin-induced hepatocarcinogenesis[31] should be confirmed in the rat liver foci assay. This assay, which has responded to 12 liver tumor promoters[26] (some of which are complete carcinogens at appropriate doses), may be particularly useful for testing the many hepatotoxic mycotoxins.

Organ-specific models may be used to assay promoting activity, supplementing the mouse skin and rat liver systems where there is sufficient evidence of organotropy. For instance, the nephrotoxin, citrinin, which has been reported to induce no tumors by itself, has enhanced dimethylnitrosamine-induced kidney tumorigenesis and has altered the spectrum of kidney tumors in rats.[32] Similarly, there is speculation that *Fusarium* toxins might play a role in the etiology of esophageal cancer.[33] This relationship might be probed by feeding the mycotoxins to rats previously initiated with a low dose of *N*-methyl-*N*-benzylnitrosamine, a specific esophageal carcinogen.[34,35] In both examples there is definite organotropy, at least a suggestion of carcinogenic activity, and a lack of bacterial mutagenicity.

IV. SCREENING MOLDY FOODS FOR CARCINOGENICITY

Human exposure to mycotoxins results primarily from ingestion of field or storage contaminated foods rather than through encounters with single pure compounds. (Bizarre exceptions have been reported or alleged, including an instance of attempted suicide with aflatoxin B_1[36] and possible chemical warfare with trichothecenes.[37]) Clearly, natural contamination of agricultural products may involve a mixture of organisms which produce a variety of toxins depending upon the substrate and its moisture content and environmental conditions such as temperature, light, and relative humidity. Furthermore, phytoalexins or chemical defense substances of plants[11] and other compounds accumulating in higher plants in response to the stress of fungal infection[12] may occur alongside mycotoxins in moldy products and even undergo further metabolic transformation by the invading fungus.[38] Since human exposure is generally to mixtures and since the toxic effects of combined exposure may differ from those caused by a single pure compound,[39-41] it is advisable to examine moldy foods, feedstuffs, or extracts thereof, as opposed to pure compounds, for carcinogenic potential.

It has been common practice to screen moldy foods or extracts of pure cultures for acute[42,44] and chronic[45,46] toxicity in rodents or domestic birds. In some such studies, known mycotoxins have accounted for less than 10% of the toxic fungal isolates.[47] A similar approach whereby moldy foods and culture extracts are screened for both initiating and promoting carcinogenic potential with microbial mutagenicity and limited in vivo cancer bioassays is advocated here. Although there have been few studies on mutagenicity screening of moldy foods or culture extracts,[48-50] such studies have revealed unique mutagenic mycotoxins elaborated by *Aspergillus chevalieri*,[51] *Alternaria alternata*,[52] and *Fusarium moniliforme*.[53] Pertinent experience in sample preparation and mutagenicity screening has come from studies on beverages,[54] home-made apple brandies,[55] and pickled vegetables[35] as well as artificial mixtures.[56] There has been little comparable application of well-defined in vivo cancer bioassays to distinguish initiating and promoting activity of moldy foods.

V. SUMMARY

Doll and Peto[1] have attributed a high proportion of cancer deaths to dietary factors. The significance of mold in these diet-related cancers cannot be fully appreciated without consideration of possible mechanisms of carcinogenesis and application of modern toxicological screening procedures not only to purified mycotoxins but more importantly to the investigation of contaminated foods and feedstuffs.

REFERENCES

1. **Doll, R. and Peto, R.,** The causes of cancer: quantitative estimates of avoidable risks of cancer in the United States today, *J. Natl. Cancer Inst.,* 66, 1191, 1981.
2. **Farber, E.,** Chemical carcinogenesis: a biologic perspective, *Am. J. Pathol.,* 106, 269, 1982.
3. **Pitot, H. C.,** The natural history of neoplastic development: the relation of experimental models to human cancer, *Cancer,* 49, 1206, 1982.
4. **Campbell, T. C.,** Chemical carcinogens and human risk assessment, *Fed. Proc. Fed. Am. Soc. Exp. Biol.,* 39, 2467, 1980.
5. **Clayson, D. B.,** Carcinogens and carcinogenesis enhancers, *Mutat. Res.,* 86, 217, 1981.
6. **Schoental, R.,** Carcinogenic mycotoxins, in *Dietary Influences on Cancer: Traditional and Modern,* Schoental, R. and Connors, T. A., Eds., CRC Press, Boca Raton, Fla., 1981, 109.
7. **Newberne, P. M. and Rogers, A. E.,** Animal toxicity of major environmental mycotoxins, in *Mycotoxins and N-Nitroso Compounds,* Vol. 1., Shank, R. C., Ed., CRC Press, Boca Raton, Fla., 1981, 51.
8. **Stark, A. A.,** Mutagenicity and carcinogenicity of mycotoxins: DNA binding as a possible mode of action, *Annu. Rev. Microbiol.,* 34, 235, 1980.
9. **Hayes, A. W.,** *Mycotoxin Teratogenicity and Mutagenicity,* CRC Press, Boca Raton, Fla., 1981, 83.
10. **Wehner, F. C., Thiel, P. G., Van Rensburg, S. J., and Demasius, I. P. C.,** Mutagenicity to *Salmonella typhimurium* of some Aspergillus and Penicillium mycotoxins, *Mutat. Res.,* 58, 193, 1978.
11. **Kuc, J.,** Compounds accumulating in plants after infection, in *Microbial Toxins,* Vol. 8, Kadis, S., Ciegler, A., and Ajl, S. J., Eds., Academic Press, New York, 1972, 211.
12. **Grisebach, H. and Ebel, J.,** Phytoalexins, chemical defense substances of higher plants? *Angew. Chem. Int. Ed. Engl.,* 17, 635, 1978.
13. **Grekin, D. A. and Epstein, J. H.,** Yearly review: psoralens, UVA (PUVA) and photocarcinogenesis, *Photochem. Photobiol.,* 33, 957, 1981.
14. **Schimmer, O. and Fischer, K.,** Metabolic inactivation of 8-methoxypsoralen (8-MOP) by rat-liver microsomal preparations, *Mutat. Res.,* 79, 327, 1980.
15. **Bridges, B. A., Greaves, M., Polani, P. E., and Wald, N.,** Do treatments available for psoriasis patients carry a genetic or carcinogenic risk? *Mutat. Res.,* 86, 279, 1981.
16. **Richards, D. E.,** The isolation and identification of toxic coumarins, in *Microbial Toxins,* Vol. 8, Kadis, S., Ciegler, A., and Ajl, S. J., Eds., Academic Press, New York, 1972, 3.
17. **Cohen, A. J.,** Critical review of the toxicology of coumarin with special reference to interspecies differences in metabolism and hepatotoxic response and their significance to man, *Food. Cosmet. Toxicol.,* 17, 277, 1979.
18. **Stoltz, D. R. and Scott, P. M.,** Mutagenicity of coumarin and related compounds for *Salmonella typhimurium, Can. J. Genet. Cytol.,* 22, 679, 1980.
19. National Toxicology Program, Mutagenesis testing results, NTP Technical Bulletin, U.S. Government Printing Office, Washington, D.C., 1(3), 10, 1980.
20. **Ciegler, A., Burmeister, H. R., Vesonder, R. F., and Hesseltine, C. W.,** Mycotoxins: occurrence in the environment, in *Mycotoxins and N-Nitroso Compounds,* Vol. 1, Shank, R. C., Ed., CRC Press, Boca Raton, Fla., 1981, 1.
21. **Hollstein, M., McCann, J., Angelosanto, F. A., and Nichols, W. W.,** Short-term tests for carcinogens and mutagens, *Mutat. Res.,* 65, 133, 1979.
22. **Weisburger, J. H. and Williams, G. M.,** Carcinogen testing: current problems and new approaches, *Science,* 214, 401, 1981.
23. **Becci, P. J., Hess, F. G., Johnson, W. D., Gallo, M. A., Babish, J. G., Dailey, R. E., and Parent, R. A.,** Long-term carcinogenicity and toxicity studies of patulin in the rat, *J. Appl. Toxicol.,* 1, 256, 1981.
24. **Tomatis, L.,** The value of long-term testing for the implementation of primary prevention, in *Origins of Human Cancer, Book C, Human Risk Assessment,* Hiatt, H. H., Watson, J. D., and Winsten, J. A., Eds., Cold Spring Harbor Laboratory, Cold Spring Harbor, N.Y., 1977, 1339.
25. **Pereira, M. A.,** Mouse skin bioassay for chemical carcinogens, *J. Am. Coll. Toxicol.,* 1, 47, 1982a.
26. **Pereira, M. A.,** Rat liver foci bioassay, *J. Am. Coll. Toxicol.,* 1, 100, 1982b.
27. **Farber, E. and Tsuda, H.,** Induction of a resistant preneoplastic liver cell as a new principle for a short-term assay *in vivo* for carcinogens, in *Short-Term Tests for Chemical Carcinogens,* Stich, H. F. and San, R. H. C., Eds., Springer-Verlag, New York, 1981, 372.
28. **Lindenfelser, L. A., Lillehoj, E. B., and Burmeister, H. R.,** Aflatoxin and trichothecene toxins: skin tumor induction and synergistic acute toxicity in white mice, *J. Natl. Cancer Inst.,* 52, 113, 1974.
29. **Roe, F. J. C. and Salaman, M. H.,** Further studies on incomplete carcinogenesis: triethylene melamine (T.E.M.), 1,2 benzanthracene and betapropiolactone as initiators of skin tumour formation in the mouse, *Br. J. Cancer,* 9, 177, 1955.

30. **Marasas, W. F. O., Bamburg, J. R., Smalley, E. B., Strong, F. M., Ragland, W. L., and Degurse, P. E.,** Toxic effects on trout, rats, and mice of T-2 toxin produced by the fungus *Fusarium tricinctum* (Cd.) Snyd. et Hans., *Toxicol. Appl. Pharmacol.*, 15, 471, 1969.

31. **Kanisawa, M. and Suzuki, S.,** Induction of renal and hepatic tumors in mice by ochratoxin A, a mycotoxin, *Gann*, 69, 599, 1978.

32. **Shinohara, Y., Arai, M., Hirao, K., Sugihara, S., Nakanishi, K., Tsuroda, H., and Ito, N.,** Combination effect of citrinin and other chemicals on rat kidney tumorigenesis, *Gann*, 67, 147, 1976.

33. **Schoental, R.,** Carcinogenic contaminants of food, in *Dietary Influences on Cancer: Traditional and Modern*, Schoental, R. and Connors, T. A., Eds., CRC Press, Boca Raton, Fla., 1981, 149.

34. **Stinson, S. F.,** Animal model: esophageal carcinoma in the rat induced with methyl-alkyl-nitrosamines, *Am. J. Pathol.*, 96, 871, 1979.

35. **Lu, S. H., Camus, A. M., Tomatis, L., and Bartsch, H.,** Mutagenicity of extracts of pickled vegetables collected in Linhsien County, a high-incidence area for esophageal cancer in Northern China, *J. Natl. Cancer Inst.*, 66, 33, 1981.

36. **Willis, R. M., Mulvihill, J. J., and Hoofnagle, J. H.,** Attempted suicide with purified aflatoxin, *Lancet*, 1, 1198, 1980.

37. **Wade, N.,** Toxin warfare charges may be premature, *Science*, 214, 34, 1981.

38. **Boyd, M. R., Dutcher, J. S., Buckpitt, A. R., Jones, R. B., and Statham, C. N.,** Role of metabolic activation in extrahepatic target organ alkylation and cytotoxicity by 4-ipomeanol, a furan derivative from moldy sweet potatoes: possible implications for carcinogenesis, in *Naturally Occurring Carcinogens-Mutagens and Modulators of Carcinogenesis*, Miller, E. C., Miller, J. A., Hirono, I., Sugimura, T., and Takayama, S., Eds., University Park Press, Baltimore, 1979, 35.

39. **Jackson, E. W., Wolf, H., and Sinnhuber, R. O.,** The relationship of hepatoma in rainbow trout to aflatoxin contamination and cottonseed meal, *Cancer Res.*, 28, 987, 1968.

40. **Wogan, G. N., Edwards, G. S., and Newberne, P. M.,** Acute and chronic toxicity of rubratoxin B, *Toxicol. Appl. Pharmacol.*, 19, 712, 1971.

41. **Sansing, G. A., Lillehoj, E. B., Detroy, R. W., and Miller, M. A.,** Synergistic toxic effects of citrinin, ochratoxin A and penicillic acid in mice, *Toxicon*, 14, 213, 1976.

42. **Kriek, N. P. J., Marasas, W. F. O., and Thiel, P. G.,** Hepato and cardiotoxicity of *Fusarium verticilloides* (*F. moniliforme*) isolates from Southern African maize, *Food Cosmet. Toxicol.*, 19, 447, 1981.

43. **Kriek, N. P. J. and Wehner, F. C.,** Toxicity of *Penicillium italicum* to laboratory animals, *Food Cosmet. Toxicol.*, 19, 311, 1981.

44. **Christensen, C. M., Nelson, G. H., Mirocha, C. J., and Bates, F.,** Toxicity to experimental animals of 943 isolates of fungi, *Cancer Res.*, 28, 2293, 1968.

45. **Frank, H. K., Orth, R., Ivankovic, S., Kuhlmann, M., and Schmähl, D.,** Investigations on carcinogenic effects of *Penicillium caseicolum* and *P. roqueforti* in rats, *Experientia*, 33, 515, 1977.

46. **Enomoto, M. and Saito, M.,** Carcinogens produced by fungi, *Annu. Rev. Microbiol.*, 26, 279, 1972.

47. **Bullerman, L. B.,** Public health significance of molds and mycotoxins in fermented dairy products, *J. Dairy Sci.*, 64, 2439, 1981.

48. **Bjeldanes, L. F., Chang, G. W., and Thomson, S. V.,** Detection of mutagens produced by fungi with the *Salmonella typhimurium* assay, *Appl. Environ. Microbiol.*, 35, 1150, 1978.

49. **Bjeldanes, L. F. and Thomson, S. V.,** Mutagenic activity of *Fusarium moniliforme* isolates in the *Salmonella typhimurium* assay, *Appl. Environ. Microbiol.*, 37, 1118, 1979.

50. **Harwig, J., Scott, P. M., Stoltz, D. R., and Blanchfield, B. J.,** Toxins of molds from decaying tomato fruits, *Appl. Environ. Microbiol.*, 38, 267, 1979.

51. **Bachmann, M., Lutby, J., and Schlatter, C.,** Toxicity and mutagenicity of molds of the *Aspergillus glaucus* group. Identification of physcion and three related anthraquinones as main toxic constituents from *Aspergillus chevalieri*, *J. Agric. Food Chem.*, 27, 1342, 1979.

52. **Scott, P. M. and Stoltz, D. R.,** Mutagens produced by *Alternaria alternata*, *Mutat. Res.*, 78, 33, 1980.

53. **Wiebe, L. A. and Bjeldanes, L. F.,** Fusarin C, a mutagen from *Fusarium moniliforme* grown on corn, *J. Food Sci.*, 46, 1424, 1981.

54. **Stoltz, D. R., Stavric, B., Krewski, D., Klassen, R., Bendall, R., and Junkins, B.,** Mutagenicity screening of foods. I. Results with beverages, *Environ. Mutagenesis*, 4, 477, 1982.

55. **Loquet, C., Toussaint, G., and LeTalaer, J. Y.,** Studies on mutagenic constituents of apple brandy and various alcoholic beverages collected in Western France, a high incidence area for esophageal cancer, *Mutat. Res.*, 88, 155, 1981.

56. **Stoltz, D. R.,** Detection of cocarcinogens and anticarcinogens with microbial mutagenicity assays, in *Short-Term Tests for Chemical Carcinogens*, Stich, H. F. and San, R. H. C., Eds., Springer-Verlag, New York, 1981, 438.

57. **Uraguchi, K., Saito, M., Noguchi, Y., Takahashi, K., Enomoto, M., and Tatsuno, T.,** Chronic toxicity and carcinogenicity in mice of the purified mycotoxins, luteoskyrin and cyclochlorotine, *Food Cosmet. Toxicol.*, 10, 193, 1972.

58. **Schoental, R., Joffe, A. Z., and Yagen, B.,** Cardiovascular lesions and various tumors found in rats given T-2 toxin, a trichothecene metabolite of *Fusarium, Cancer Res.,* 39, 2179, 1979.

59. National Toxicology Program, Carcinogenesis bioassay results, NTP Technical Bulletin, U.S. Government Printing Office, Washington, D.C., 6, 7, 1982.

60. **Schoental, R.,** Role of podophyllotoxin in the bedding and dietary zearalenone on incidence of spontaneous tumors in laboratory animals, *Cancer Res.,* 34, 2419, 1974.

61. **Moule, Y., Decloitre, F., and Hamon, G.,** Mutagenicity of the mycotoxin botryodiplodin in the *Salmonella typhimurium*/microsomal activation test, *Environ. Mutagenesis,* 3, 287, 1981.

62. **Brown, J. P. and Brown, R. J.,** Mutagenesis by 9,10-anthraquinone derivatives and related compounds in *Salmonella typhimurium, Mutat. Res.,* 40, 203, 1976.

63. **Bjeldanes, L. F. and Chew, H.,** Mutagenicity of 1,2-dicarbonyl compounds: maltol, kojic acid, diacetyl and related substances, *Mutat. Res.,* 67, 367, 1979.

64. **Stark, A. A., Townsend, J. M., Wogan, G. N., Demain, A. L., Manmade, A., and Ghosh, A. C.,** Mutagenicity and antibacterial activity of mycotoxins produced by *P. islandicum* Sopp. and *P. rugulosum, J. Environ. Pathol. Toxicol.,* 2, 313, 1978.

65. **Stark, A. A., Kobbe, B., Matsuo, K., Buchi, G., Wogan, G. N., and Demain, A. L.,** Mollicellins: mutagenic and antibacterial mycotoxins, *Appl. Environ. Microbiol.,* 36, 412, 1978.

Chapter 14

MUTAGENIC ACTIVITY OF DRINKING WATER

Earle Nestmann

TABLE OF CONTENTS

I. INTRODUCTION

Municipal drinking water is usually supplied by nearby rivers or lakes which contain varying amounts of natural and anthropogenic organic compounds from varied sources (e.g., agriculture, industry, urban centers). Many of the compounds (e.g., halogenated and many other oxidized compounds) in finished (treated) drinking water probably are formed by reactions of the constituents of the untreated water with chlorine during disinfection.[1] Certain of these compounds (e.g., dichloromethane, chloroform) are known to be mutagenic and/ or carcinogenic in experimental organisms at doses many thousands of times greater than levels to which man is exposed through the water supply. However, it is not practical to test all known constituents of drinking water for possible toxic effects, or even to identify every contaminant present in trace amounts. Consequently, attempts are underway to study the toxic potential of drinking water by testing concentrates or extracts. Due to the small quantities of organic material in these extracts, sensitive test methods are required. Many research investigations of organic extracts have involved bacterial mutagenicity tests. Recent studies have shown that organic extracts of chlorinated,[2-7] ozonated,[2] and untreated[8] drinking water samples from diverse locations throughout the world are mutagenic in the *Salmonella/ mammalian-microsome assay.*[9] Extracts of drinking water are complex mixtures of organics and, thus, the study of their biological effects is subject to different approaches and interpretation in comparison to the testing of individual compounds.[1,10] The research and literature on drinking water mutagenicity published prior to 1980 was reviewed comprehensively by Loper.[1] The purpose of this review is to summarize the more recent literature and to discuss the observations reported.

II. REVIEW OF METHODS AND FINDINGS

A. Concentrated Samples
1. Macroreticular Resin Extraction
One of the most widely adopted methods for concentrating certain of the dilute organics present in drinking water is adsorption on XAD macroreticular resins. These adsorbents can be conveniently used in laboratory or field studies by preparing cartridges for connection to taps or pumps which supply water at constant flow rates for periods of sampling.[11] Some of the most extensive recent surveys of the mutagenicity of drinking water were performed on Canadian water supplies using XAD-2 resins[2,3] and on Dutch water using a combination of XAD-4/8 resins.[12] Both methods appear to be suitable for concentrating mutagenic contaminants of drinking water.

Using the methods and strategies for sampling and mutagenicity testing developed in an earlier pilot study (200 ℓ samples concentrated 2 to 5 $\times$ 10^4 times; strains TA98 and TA100; $\pm$ S9),[8] a survey involving water supplies of 29 municipalities (30 treatment plants) throughout Canada was undertaken.[2] Mutagenicity in *Salmonella* was found for all communities in the study (Table 1), however, due to seasonal variations in mutagenic potency that also had been noted previously[8] and later,[13-16] sampling in both winter and summer seasons was required for detection of mutagenic activity in certain municipalities. Metabolic activation by S9 reduced the mutagenic responses, and strain TA100 was far more sensitive than TA98 in detecting mutagenic activity. However, for 6 of the 90 extracts tested in both strains, mutagenicity was found only in strain TA98. Data from one representative sample are shown in Figure 1. Tests were performed on both liquid (XAD eluent reduced to 10 mℓ 15% acetone/hexane) and solid (XAD eluent reduced to dryness and dissolved in dimethyl sulfoxide) extracts due to concern about possible interaction of the test material with dimethyl sulfoxide.[17] A comparison of the initial slopes of the dose-effect curves for the liquid and solid extracts in Figure 1 shows little or no difference, which probably means an absence

Table 1
SUMMARY OF CANADIAN STUDIES ON THE
MUTAGENICITY OF DRINKING WATER EXTRACTS

Treatment plant[a]	Source[b]	Winter[c]	Summer[c]	Ref.
St. John's, N.F.	L	165	684	2
Amherst, N. S.	W			8
Dartmouth, N. S.,	L	581	689	2
Halifax, N.S.	L	360	659	2
Truro, N. S.	L	771	853	2
Fredericton, N.B.	W	279	526	2
Saint John, N.B.	L	95	1792	2
Drummondville, Q.	R	727	355	2
Granby, Q.	R	779	228	2
Montréal-Lasalle, Q.	R	369	776	2
Laval, Q.	R	652	666	2
Longueuil, Q.	R	458	428	2
Quebec City-Loretteville	R,L	161	951	2
Amherstburg, O.	R	170	801	3
Amherstburg, O.	R	170	801	3
Barrie, O.	W	213	508	2
Brantford, O.	R	165	1140	2
Brockville, O.	R			8
Goderich, O.	L	289	816	3
Guelph, O.	W	146	260	2
Kingston, O.	L	201	442	3
Ottawa-Brittania, O.	R	684	857	2,8
Ottawa-Lemieux Isl., O.	R	686	677	2,8
Owen Sound, O.	L	410	674	3
Perth, O.,	R			8
Port Colbourne, O.	L	370	897	3
Port Dover, O.	L	350	1154	3
Prescott, O.	R			8
St. Catharines, O.	L	192	705	3
Sarnia, O.	L	164	763	3
Sault Ste. Marie, O.	R	180	188	3
Smiths Falls, O.	R			8
Sudbury, O.	R	1377	1001	2
Thunder Bay, O.	L	240,512	505,521	2,3
Toronto, O.	L	360,688	586,455	2,3
Union/Leamington, O.	L	149	970	3
Selkirk, M.	R	140	559	2
Winnipeg, M.	L	300	709	2
Regina, S.	L	388	574	2
Saskatoon, S.	R	298	230	2
Calgary, A.	L,R	422	533	2
Edmonton, A.	R	175	219	2
Medicine Hat, A.	R	158	577	2
Kelowna, B.C.	L	357	293	2
Penticton, B.C.	R	634	1283	2
Vancouver, B.C.	L	228	414	2

[a] Treatment plant locations arranged geographically by province, East to West, and alphabetically within each province. Abbreviations: N.F., Newfoundland; N.S., Nova Scotia; N.B., New Brunswick; Q, Québec; O, Ontario; M, Manitoba; S, Saskatchewan; A, Alberta; B.C., British Columbia.

[b] Type of water source: L, lake; R, river; W, well.

[c] Maximal responses in strain TA100 for dry extract (revertants/plate) values for early study not tabulated since samples were taken in spring and fall.

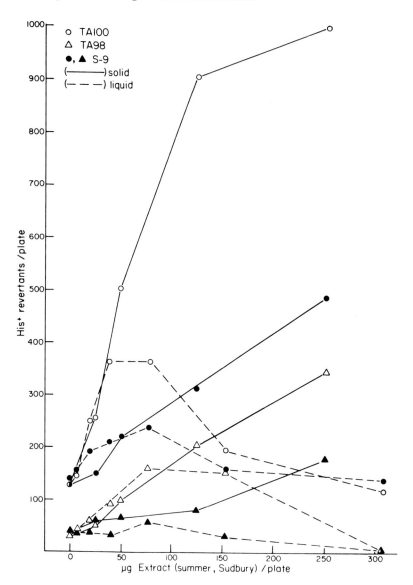

FIGURE 1.   Mutagenicity in *Salmonella* strains TA98 and TA100 (± S9) with exposure to solid (XAD-2 eluent taken to dryness and dissolved in DMSO) and liquid (concentrated acetone/hexane XAD-2 eluent) extracts of a summer sample of Sudbury, Ontario, drinking water.

of interaction of the solid extract with DMSO. As doses were increased, however, the curves diverged due to the toxic effect of the solvent (acetone/hexane) in the liquid extract. In certain other cases, the initial slopes do not overlap (data not shown), indicating that choice of solvent does contribute to the pattern of extract mutagenicity observed. In addition, Grabow et al.[16] observed that water extracts in DMSO induced significantly reduced mutagenicity after storage for 2 to 3 days at 4°C. These findings emphasize the importance of being cognizant of possible solvent effects.[17]

Another survey involved samples taken at 12 Canadian municipalities using the Great Lakes system as their source of drinking water.[3] Most of the general conclusions were the same as for the previous study[2] regarding the seasonal variation, the more sensitive tester strain, and the deactivating effects of S9. Since drinking water from the Great Lakes has

Table 2
AVERAGE MAXIMAL
RESPONSES FOR TREATMENT
PLANTS WITH DIFFERENT
TYPES OF WATER SOURCES

Type of water[a]	Revertants/plate (±S.D.)	
	Winter	**Summer**
River	478 (340)	624 (340)
Lake	341 (178)	721 (318)
Wells	212 (66)	431 (149)

[a]   Number of treatment plants for each category:
rivers, 16; lakes, 21; wells, 3.

been reported to contain levels of anthropogenic compounds lower than those found in drinking water from river sources,[18,19] comparisons of mutagenic potencies were made amongst three types of water (river, lake, well) sampled in the two surveys.[2,3] Exact quantitative comparisons are difficult to justify because of complex responses in bacterial mutagenicity after exposure to mixtures, however, the methods of sampling, extract preparation, and mutagenicity testing were identical in both studies, thereby reducing possible errors due to these variables. Shown in Table 2 are the means (± S.D.) of the maximal responses in strain TA100 for all treatment plants drawing water exclusively from a river, lake, or well source. Although the responses vary considerably within these sub-groupings, certain generalizations can be made. Average mutagenicity of the extracts was higher in the summer samples for each of the three water source types, and the mutagenic activity found in concentrates of organics from well water was lower compared to river or lake sources. No consistent difference in the mutagenicity of extracts was apparent between rivers and lakes since the former showed a higher average in the winter and a lower average in the summer. The same pattern was found when the Great Lakes sources were considered separately and compared to river sources (not shown). Therefore, the higher levels of certain organics measured in rivers (compared to the Great Lakes)[18,19] could be related to the higher mutagenic responses from winter's extracts but not from summer's extracts. A similar comparison of 18 cities in The Netherlands also has been made, but the types of water sources were different.[12,13]

Comprehensive studies by Kool et al.[20,21] compared a number of variations in sample collection and preparation to determine a reliable standard method for surface and drinking waters in The Netherlands. For this comparative study, surface water was concentrated by factors of 1 to 7×10^3, and chlorinated drinking water prepared from the rivers Rhine and Meuse was concentrated 6×10^3-fold. No difference in mutagenic activity was found between XAD-2 resin and a mixture of XAD-4/8, and the investigators elected to use XAD-4/8. Comparing solvents acetone and DMSO for elution of the columns, DMSO was preferred since direct testing of volumes up to 0.5 mℓ was possible and an evaporation step with acetone was eliminated. The amount of solvent required to elute most of the mutagenic compounds from the column was equivalent to the amount of resin in the column (bed volume). For surface and drinking waters (both nonchlorinated), TA98 was found to be a more sensitive indicator of mutagenic activity than TA100, in contrast to findings for chlorinated drinking water.[2,3,8] Extracts of surface and drinking waters showed nearly equivalent mutagenicity without S9. The presence of S9 enhanced the mutagenicity of surface water extracts but reduced the activity found in drinking water, the general pattern found for most drinking water samples.[2,3,5,6,8,12] This deactivation of extract mutagenicity is not surprising in view of the observations that certain individual chlorinated compounds found in drinking water (and in pulp mill effluent) show the same pattern of mutagenicity reduction with S9.[22,23]

In addition to assaying whole extracts for mutagenicity, efforts are underway to identify specific mutagens present in drinking water. Using HPLC fractionation, a direct acting mutagen in strain TA98 has been isolated from an extract of a large U.S. drinking water sample, and preliminary analysis seems to indicate a nonchlorinated compound whose MS does not correspond with NIH/EPA data base entries.[24] Other investigators have studied the presence of many organic compounds in connection with different water treatment strategies in The Netherlands.[6] Treatments appear to introduce some types of compounds and/or break down others, and identification of several has been possible.

Test systems other than *Salmonella* have been used in mutagenicity studies of drinking water. XAD-2 columns were used to prepare extracts of Illinois drinking water for a study involving four short-term tests (*Salmonella, Neurospora crassa, Saccharomyces cerevisiae,* and *Zea mays*). Nearly all the extracts were nonmutagenic, but they were concentrated by a factor of only 250. In studies of recycled water samples from advanced treatment plants, positive effects were found in *Salmonella* strain TA100 with XAD-8 extracts,[26] ouabain-resistant mutants were induced in Chinese hamster V79 cells (with S9), and transformants were induced in WI-38 human embryonic lung cells.[27] In the latter study, transformants were not induced by positive control compounds N-methyl-N'-nitro-N-nitrosoguanidine or benzo[a]pyrene. It was suggested that this was due to the absence of a promotor which likely would be present in the complex mixture (which had been concentrated 1000-fold by reverse osmosis). A similar extract had been reported previously by these authors to be nonmutagenic in *Salmonella*.[27] Concentrates of volatile and nonvolatile components of drinking water induced no teratogenic effects in progeny of treated pregnant mice.[28]

2. Liquid-Liquid Extraction

Liquid-liquid extraction of organic compounds from certain aqueous mixtures and suspensions (e.g., activated sludge effluents) may be the preferred method of concentration due to the presence of particulate matter. Not only can particles block adsorption columns, but the liquid-liquid extraction removes compounds adsorbed to this matter. This was the experimental rationale in a South African study[29] in which it was found that samples taken at various stages in a water reclamation plant became less mutagenic in *Salmonella* after ferric chloride clarification (with interstage chlorination). No detectable mutagenicity was found after further chemical breakdown with ozonation or after final chlorination of this highly oxidized material.[29] The same method of extraction (dichloromethane) also proved to be useful in the detection of mutagenicity in secondary treated wastewater effluents and in samples of the Vaal River (South Africa) below the point of receiving residential and industrial discharges, but it was less effective in the evaluation of Pretoria drinking water.[4] A similar extraction (dichloromethane) was performed in a Belgian study on the River Meuse,[30] and as with the two previous studies,[4,29] most mutagenic activity was found only in the presence of metabolic activation (S9) in *Salmonella* strains TA1538 and TA98, which revert by frameshift mutations.[9] Water samples from 7 sites along the Sava River in Yugoslavia were extracted with hexane and tested for mutagenicity using only one strain (TA100), and one sample showed a mutagenic response which required S9.[31] A combination of extraction by petroleum ether and separation and concentration steps using chemical and chromatographic methods[32] was used to show that extracts of the water from the Rhine induced base substitution mutations in *Salmonella* strain TA100 (the only strain used) with or without S9.[33] In all these studies, the extracted organics were concentrated by evaporation of the solvent to dryness, and the residues were dissolved in DMSO for testing in bacteria. Possible solvent-extract interactions were not considered.

3. *Comparisons of Concentration Procedures*

Grabow et al.[34] performed an extensive study comparing the relative abilities of liquid-liquid extraction (with dichloromethane) and XAD (-2 and -7) resin to concentrate organics with detectable mutagenic activity in repeated samples of reclaimed water, drinking water, and raw river water. Water samples (100 ℓ) were concentrated by factors of 2 to 5×10^4, and in most cases (20 of 26), the dichloromethane-extracted material showed higher mutagenic activity than XAD extracts. The authors pointed out, however, that recovery efficiency for different mutagens could vary, and XAD-2 may be more efficient for mutagens at very low concentrations.[34] Studies[5,34] have shown that preparation of extracts using XAD-7, for concentrating organics not first adsorbed by XAD-2, does not seem to help significantly in the detection of mutagenic activity of water samples.

In another study,[35] selective adsorption of organics by XAD-2 was compared with freeze drying as an alternate method of nonselectively concentrating material in water samples. It was found that the volumes of water required to find a mutagenic response were usually slightly lower with freeze drying, but the patterns of response were similar with both methods.[35] A difficulty with the freeze drying method may arise when relatively large amounts of natural organics (e.g., humic and fulvic acids) are present. These and other nonmutagenic compounds in the freeze-dried samples, which would not be present in XAD extracts, may contribute to sample insolubility and perhaps toxicity in the test organism.

B. Unconcentrated Samples

Modifications of the *Salmonella*/mammalian-microsome assay for testing unconcentrated water were reviewed by Loper.[1] Kool et al.[20] have stated that, since the mutagens and carcinogens known to be in river water are present at such low concentrations ($\mu g/\ell$), testing of unconcentrated water in *Salmonella* would not be expected to show mutagenic effects. The marginal results reported may be subject to variables affecting growth of the tester strains.[20]

A more sensitive test, the modified fluctuation assay devised by Green et al.,[36] has been used with *Salmonella* strains to determine whether it can be used reliably to study the mutagenic potential of unconcentrated drinking water. An initial study reported that only weak responses were observed which possibly could be due to artefacts of bacterial growth.[35] Subsequently, in more detailed studies using the fluctuation procedure, most of the positive responses found were shown to be artefactual.[37,38]

Other studies concerned with unconcentrated water have involved cytogenetic effects in the Eastern Mudminnow *(Umbra pygmaea)* of untreated water from the river Rhine.[33,39,40] These fish, exposed to the Rhine's water for different lengths of time, showed increased chromosome breaks and sister chromatid exchanges in their gill cells. Unconcentrated water from the Rhine was not tested in *Salmonella* in these studies, and a conclusion about the relative sensitivity of the fish and bacterial assays cannot be drawn. It appears, however, that the Mudminnow assay could be a useful monitoring method for unconcentrated water. In one of these studies,[33] accompanying *Salmonella* tests were performed on extracts of the same water with positive effects for the aromatic hydrocarbon fraction.

Collins et al.[41] undertook a study of reservoir water after an epidemiological investigation found that a high birth defect rate was associated with its consumption. Repeated samples of filter-sterilized, unconcentrated water were tested throughout the year, and three samples were found to induce two- and threefold increases of revertant colonies in *Salmonella*. Positive effects were found only in strain TA1537 (showing a high spontaneous background) with S9 pre-incubation, and these responses were correlated with algal blooms in the reservoir. Another year of sampling showed no mutagenic responses, but also no algal bloom. Homogenized laboratory cultures of the predominant alga were nonmutagenic. A pilot rat reproductive study was initiated at the time of the algal bloom, and a genetically transmitted neurological abnormality was observed which was not found in subsequent litters that were exposed to nonmutagenic water. The mutagenic water also showed ichthyotoxicity to *Gambusia affinis*, but nonmutagenic reservoir water was not tested. The inference from this study is that algal toxins, produced in sufficient quantity in drinking water, may be responsible for genetic and toxic effects in a variety of target organisms.[41]

III. EFFECTS OF WATER TREATMENT

A comparison of the mutagenic activity of water extracts, before and following disinfection, shows that chlorination usually leads to an increase in mutagenicity.[1,8] More recent studies show that this appears to be a consistent trend. Examination of the mutagenicity of liquid-extracted organics from unchlorinated and chlorinated samples of lake, river, and ground waters indicated that extracts of ground water showed no mutagenic effects with or without chlorination; lake water showed a response only after chlorination and river water showed a higher mutagenic response after chlorination. The mutagenic activity of the water samples was related to their chemical oxygen demands representing the approximate quantity of organic compounds present which could react with the chlorine.[7] Another study[2] found that total organic carbon did not correlate highly with mutagenic activity of extracts of chlorinated water in *Salmonella*. Chlorination during advanced treatment of wastewater also strongly enhanced the mutagenicity of the water extract (concentrated by XAD-8).[26] A heavily polluted river was subjected to a study in which the chemicals in the water were concentrated (XAD-2) after different types of treatment. Extracts of water which was untreated or treated only with coagulants showed a low degree of mutagenicity in strain TA1538, the strain determined to be the most sensitive with initial concentrates. Extracts of chlorinated water, with or without coagulation, showed much higher mutagenic responses.[42]

These reports support the need to study alternate methods of disinfection. Certain Canadian water treatment plants disinfect with ozone, but the water is also post-chlorinated to establish a chlorine residual for distribution. Extracts of these supplies show mutagenic responses in *Salmonella*.[2] When humic and fulvic acids, naturally present in water supplies, are chlorinated, they are known to produce measurable levels of trihalomethane compounds and other chlorinated organics. The mutagenicity of ozonated soil fulvic acid is very weak[43] and is enhanced with subsequent chlorination.[44] On the other hand, in a Belgian pilot plant which treated prechlorinated water with different doses of ozone, the mutagenic activity (in XAD-2 extracts) of the chlorinated influent detectable by strain TA98 was eliminated and the activity found using strain TA100 was reduced in a dose-dependent manner.[45] In another study,[12] the weak mutagenicity of raw water extracts (XAD-4/8) from the river Meuse at one Dutch city was only slightly reduced (with S9) with ozonation, completely eliminated with activated carbon filtration ($\pm$S9), but partially restored in the finished water after post-chlorination. Extracts from another city drawing water from the Meuse showed that a combination of dune infiltration, slow sand filtration and activated carbon (powder) filtration removed all the mutagenicity that was found in the raw and transport-chlorinated water samples.[12]

Other methods of water disinfection include ammonia/chlorine processes (chloramination) which is one of the more widely practiced alternate schemes in use, but little is known about its effects on mutagenicity or other toxicological endpoints.[46] The most comprehensive comparison of the mutagenicity associated with the by-products of different types of disinfection methods appears to be a Dutch study concerning chlorine, chlorine dioxide, ozone, and UV-irradiation.[6] Although the extent of mutagenicity of XAD-4/8 extracts was different for the two rivers studied (Meuse and Rhine), in general, treatments by chlorine and chlorine dioxide enhanced mutagenic activity, ozonation reduced it, and UV-irradiation had no effect. In addition, ozone was the most effective in the removal of compounds identified in raw water. This study also examined the identity of compounds formed by the disinfection processes, and it was found that chlorination, but not chlorine dioxide treatment, leads to the formation of trihalomethanes. Since the mutagenicity was enhanced by both processes to similar extents, this may be interpreted to mean that trihalomethane formation was not correlated with this particular form of toxicity.[6] In agreement with this finding, another study found that unchlorinated volatile compounds in treated drinking water (e.g., ethyl benzene, toluene, and xylenes) were more highly correlated with the mutagenic activity of XAD-2 extracts of the water than were trihalomethanes.[2]

IV. CONCLUSIONS

Most extracts of chlorinated drinking water and many extracts of other types of water are mutagenic in the *Salmonella*/mammalian-microsome assay. Different methods for concentrating samples appear to be particularly well suited to different sources of water. In addition, the extent to which samples have been concentrated varies among studies in the literature. The diverse sources of water (i.e., extent of contamination), treatments, the varied methods for concentration, as well as the extent of concentration of samples, are partially responsible for the different responses reported. Another factor is the choice of bacterial strain(s) for testing. Several studies have employed five strains (TA1535, TA100, TA1537, TA1538, and TA98) in the *Salmonella* assay;[9] others use the two generally most sensitive strains (TA98 and TA100), which enable detection of both frameshift and base substitution mutations, and other investigators test with only one strain, sometimes with preliminary work as the basis for selection. Mutagenicity of drinking water often varies with the season of sampling, summer and early fall samples showing more activity than winter and early spring. All these variables make generalizations from the literature difficult, if not impossible.

A conservative approach to testing drinking water for mutagenicity should involve concentrating samples to produce enough material to give measurable activity in the least contaminated types of water. Sampling would be done in different seasons, and bacterial testing would include use of both strains TA98 and TA100. This is the approach used in the extensive Canadian studies[2,3,8] in which mutagenic activity was found in drinking water from 44 (of 45) different treatment plants. It is not possible to make comparisons from location to location, season to season, etc., if there is no detectable activity in many of the extracts.

Understandably, when drinking water is concentrated to the extent of 5×10^4-fold and mutagenic activity is found, the question arises concerning the meaning of these positive responses. A general interpretation is that drinking water contains trace levels of organic compounds that, when concentrated, are mutagenic in bacteria. It can be deduced that differing amounts of these compounds in the extracts can lead to different levels of mutagenic response, although it must be kept in mind that, when complex mixtures of compounds are tested, many additive, synergistic, and antagonistic interactions may take place.[10] Thus, it is not sufficient to determine analytically the levels of a few key compounds to predict the mutagenicity of a water supply, nor can it be assumed that the same interactions that occur in the *Salmonella* test will be found in another assay.[47]

It is imperative to acknowledge that screening drinking water extracts for bacterial mutagenicity is not a reliable way to determine safety or hazard of any drinking water source. At present, these must be regarded as research studies, not attempts to establish the basis for regulation.[10,20] Bacterial testing is valuable for setting priorities for further investigations, but human risk must be determined on the basis of in vivo mammalian studies.

ACKNOWLEDGMENTS

I wish to thank Drs. G. R. Douglas, G. L. LeBel, and D. H. Blakey for suggestions concerning the manuscript; Drs. D. T. Williams, R. Otson, and G. L. LeBel for their cooperation; Dr. G. C. Becking for continuing encouragement; and I. Stegner for typing.

REFERENCES

1. **Loper, J. C.,** Mutagenic effects of organic compounds in drinking water, *Mutat. Res.,* 76, 241, 1980.
2. **Nestmann, E. R., Otson, R., LeBel, G. L., Williams, D. T., Lee, E. G.-H., and Biggs, D. C.,** Correlation of water quality parameters with mutagenicity of drinking water extracts, in *Water Chlorination: Environmental Impact and Health Effects,* Vol. 4, Jolley, R. L., Brungs, W. A., Cotruvo, J. A., Cumming, R. B., Mattice, J. S., and Jacobs, V., Eds., Ann Arbor Science Publishing, Ann Arbor, Mich., 1983, 1151.
3. **Williams, D. T., Nestmann, E. R., LeBel, G. L., Benoit, F. M., and Otson, R.,** Determination of mutagenic potential and organic contaminants of Great Lakes drinking water, *Chemosphere,* 11, 263, 1982.
4. **Grabow, W. O. K., Denkhaus, R., and van Rossum, P. G.,** Detection of mutagens in wastewater, a polluted river and drinking water by means of the Ames *Salmonella*/microsome assay, *S. Afr. J. Sci.,* 76, 118, 1980.
5. **Loper, J. C., Tabor, M. W., and Miles, S. K.,** Mutagenic subfractions from nonvolatile organics of drinking water, in *Water Chlorination: Environmental Impact and Health Effects,* Vol. 4, Jolley, R. L. et al., Eds., Ann Arbor Scientific Publishing, Ann Arbor, Mich., 1983, 1199.
6. **Zoeteman, B. C. J., Hrubec, J., de Greef, E., and Kool, H. J.,** Mutagenic activity associated with by-products of drinking water disinfection by chlorine, chlorine dioxide, ozone and UV-irradiation, *Environ. Health Perspect.,* 46, 197, 1982.
7. **Maruoka, S. and Yamanaka, S.,** Production of mutagenic substances by chlorination of waters, *Mutat. Res.,* 79, 381, 1980.
8. **Nestmann, E. R., LeBel, G. L., Williams, D. T., and Kowbel, D. J.,** Mutagenicity of organic extracts from Canadian drinking water in the *Salmonella*/mammalian-microsome assay, *Environ. Mutagenesis,* 1, 337, 1979.
9. **Ames, B. N., McCann, J., and Yamasaki, E.,** Methods for detecting carcinogens and mutagens with the *Salmonella*/mammalian-microsome mutagenicity test, *Mutat. Res.,* 31, 347, 1975.
10. **Nestmann, E. R. and Douglas, G. R.,** New tools for assessing mutagenic and carcinogenic risk of municipal and industrial wastewaters, in *Advances in Biotechnology,* Vol. 2, Moo-Young, M. and Robinson, C. W., Eds., Pergamon Press, Elmsford, N.Y., 649, 1981.
11. **LeBel, G. L., Williams, D. T., Griffith, G., and Benoit, F. M.,** Isolation and concentration of organophosphorus pesticides from drinking water at the ng/L level, using macroreticular resin, *J. Assoc. Off. Anal. Chem.,* 62, 241, 1979.
12. **Kool, H. J., van Kreijl, C. F., de Greef, E., and van Kranen, H. J.,** Presence, introduction and removal of mutagenic activity during the preparation of drinking water in the Netherlands, *Environ. Health Perspect.,* 46, 207, 1982.
13. **Slooff, W. and van Kreijl, C. F.,** Monitoring the rivers Rhine and Meuse in The Netherlands for mutagenic activity using the Ames test in combination with rat or fish liver homogenates, *Aquatic Toxicol.,* 2, 89, 1982.
14. **Kool, H. J., van Kreijl, C. F., van Kranen, H. J., and de Greef, E.,** Toxicity assessment of organic compounds in drinking water in The Netherlands, *Sci. Total Environ.,* 18, 135, 1981.
15. **Grimm-Kibalo, S. M., Glatz, B. A., and Fritz, J. S.,** Seasonal variation of mutagenic activity in drinking water, *Bull. Environ. Contaminants Toxicol.,* 26, 188, 1981.
16. **Grabow, W. O. K., van Rossum, P. G., Grabow, N. A., and Denkhaus, R.,** Relationship of the raw water quality to mutagens detectable by the Ames *Salmonella*/microsome assay in a drinking water supply, *Water Res.,* 15, 1037, 1981.
17. **Nestmann, E. R., Chu, I., Kowbel, D. J., and Matula, T. I.,** Short-lived mutagen in *Salmonella* produced by reaction of trichloroacetic acid and dimethyl sulphoxide, *Can. J. Genet. Cytol.,* 22, 35, 1980.
18. Status Report on the Persistent Toxic Pollutants in the Lake Ontario Basin, International Joint Commission, Water Quality Board Report, Appendix E, Windsor, Ontario, Canada, 1976.
19. Status Report on Organic and Heavy Metal Contaminants in the Lakes Erie, Michigan, Huron and Superior Basins, International Joint Commission, Water Quality Board Report, Appendix E, Windsor, Ontario, Canada, 1978.
20. **Kool, H. J., van Kreijl, C. F., van Kranen, H. J., and de Greef, E.,** The use of XAD-resins for the detection of mutagenic activity in water. I. Studies with surface water, *Chemosphere,* 10, 85, 1981.
21. **Kool, H. J., van Kreijl, C. F., and van Kranen, H. J.,** The use of XAD-resins for the detection of mutagenic activity in water. II. Studies with drinking water, *Chemosphere,* 10, 99, 1981.
22. **Nestmann, E. R., Lee, E. G.-H., Matula, T. I., Douglas, G. R., and Mueller, J. C.,** Mutagenicity of constituents identified in pulp and paper mill effluents using the *Salmonella*/mammalian-microsome assay, *Mutat. Res.,* 79, 203, 1980.
23. **Nestmann, E. R., Otson, R., Williams, D. T., and Kowbel, D. J.,** Mutagenicity of paint removers containing dichloromethane, *Cancer Lett.,* 11, 295, 1981.

24. **Loper, J. C., Tabor, M. W., and MacDonald, S. M.,** Mutagens from non-volatile organics of drinking water, *Environ. Mutagenesis,* 4(Abstr.), 380, 1982.
25. **DeMarini, D. M., Plewa, M. J., and Brockman, H. E.,** Use of four short-term tests to evaluate the mutagenicity of municipal water, *J. Toxicol. Environ. Health,* 9, 127, 1982.
26. **Reinhard, M., Goodman, N., and Mortelmans, K.,** Occurrence of mutagenic residues in advanced treated wastewater, Fourth Conference on Water Chlorination: Environmental Impact and Health Effects, Asilomar, 1981.
27. **Gruener, N. and Lockwood, M. P.,** Mutagenicity and transformation by recycled water, *J. Toxicol. Environ. Health,* 5, 663, 1979.
28. **Kavlock, R., Chernoff, N., Carver, B., and Kopfler, F.,** Teratology studies in mice exposed to municipal drinking water concentrates during organogenesis, *Food Cosmet. Toxicol.,* 17, 343, 1979.
29. **Denkhaus, R., Grabow, W. O. K., and Prozesky, O. W.,** Removal of mutagenic compounds in a wastewater reclamation system evaluated by means of the Ames *Salmonella*/microsome assay, *Prog. Water Technol.,* 12, 571, 1980.
30. **van Hoof, F. and Verheyden, J.,** Mutagenic activity in the River Meuse in Belgium, *Sci. Total Environ.,* 20, 15, 1981.
31. **Kurelec, B., Protic, M., Britvic, S., Kezic, N., Rijavec, M., and Zahn, R. K.,** Toxic effects in fish and mutagenic capacity of water from the Sava River in Yugoslavia, *Bull. Environ. Contaminants Toxicol.,* 26, 179, 1981.
32. **Meijers, A. P. and van der Leer, R. Chr.,** The occurrence of organic micropollutants in the river Rhine and the river Maas, *Water Res.,* 10, 597, 1976.
33. **Prein, A. E., Thie, G. M., Alink, G. M., Koeman, J. H., and Poels, C. L. M.,** Cytogenetic changes in fish exposed to water of the river Rhine, *Sci. Total Environ.,* 9, 287, 1978.
34. **Grabow, W. O. K., Burger, J. S., and Hilner, C. A.,** Comparison of liquid-liquid extraction and resin adsorption for concentrating mutagens in Ames *Salmonella*/microsome assays on water, *Bull. Environ. Contaminants Toxicol.,* 27, 442, 1981.
35. **Forster, R. and Wilson, I.,** The application of mutagenicity testing to drinking water, *J. Inst. Water Eng. Sci.,* 35, 259, 1981.
36. **Green, M. H. L., Muriel, W. J., and Bridges, B. A.,** Use of a simplified fluctuation test to detect low levels of mutagens, *Mutat. Res.,* 38, 33, 1976.
37. **Forster, R., Green, M. H. L., Gwilliam, R. D., Priestly, A., and Bridges, B. A.,** The use of the fluctuation test to detect mutagenic activity in unconcentrated samples of drinking waters in the United Kingdom, in *Water Chlorination: Environmental Impact and Health Effects,* Vol. 4, Jolley, R. J., Brungs, W. A., Cotruvo, J. A., Cumming, R. B., Mattice, J. S., and Jacobs, V., Eds., Ann Arbor Science Publishing, Ann Arbor, Mich., 1983, 1189.
38. **Harrington, T. R., Nestmann, E. R., and Kowbel, D. J.,** Suitability of the modified bacterial fluctuation assay for evaluating mutagenicity of unconcentrated drinking water, *Mutat. Res.,* 120, 97, 1983.
39. **Alink, G. M., Frederix-Wolters, E. M. H., van der Gaag, M. A., van de Kerkhoff, J. F. J., and Poels, C. L. M.,** Induction of sister-chromatid exchanges in fish exposed to Rhine water, *Mutat. Res.,* 78, 369, 1980.
40. **Hooftman, R. N. and Vink, G. J.,** Cytogenetic effects on the Eastern Mudminnow, *Umbra pygmaea,* exposed to ethyl methanesulfonate, benzo(a)pyrene, and river water, *Ecotoxicol. Environ. Safety,* 5, 261, 1981.
41. **Collins, M. D., Gowans, C. S., Garro, F., Estervig, D., and Swanson, T.,** Temporal association between an algal bloom and mutagenicity in a water reservoir, in *The Water Environment: Algal Toxins and Health,* Carmichael, W. W., Ed., Plenum Press, New York, 1981, 271.
42. **Flanagan, E. P. and Allen, H. E.,** Effect of water treatment on mutagenic potential, *Bull. Environ. Contaminants Toxicol.,* 27, 765, 1981.
43. **Kowbel, D. J., Nestmann, E. R., Malaiyandi, M., and Helleur, R.,** Determination of mutagenic activity in *Salmonella* of residual fulvic acids after ozonation, *Water Res.,* 16, 1537, 1982.
44. **Kowbel, D. J., Nestmann, E. R., Paramsigamani, V., and Malaiyandi, M.,** Mutagenicity in *Salmonella* of chlorinated residues of soil fulvic acid after pretreatment with ozone, submitted.
45. **van Hoof, F.,** Influence of ozonation on direct-acting mutagens formed during drinking water chlorination, in *Water Chlorination: Environmental Impact and Health Effects,* Vol. 4, Jolly, R. J. et al., Eds., Ann Arbor Scientific Publishing, Ann Arbor, Mich., 1983, 1211.
46. **Moore, G. S. and Calabrese, E. J.,** The health effects of chloramines in potable water supplies: a literature review, *J. Environ. Pathol. Toxicol.,* 4, 257, 1980.
47. **Salamone, M. F., Heddle, J. A., Gingerich, J., and Katz, M.,** On the complexities of risk estimates, metabolic activation, and chemical mixtures, in *Progress in Mutation Research,* Vol. 3, Bora, K. C., Douglas, G. R., and Nestmann, E. R., Eds., Elsevier, Amsterdam, 179, 1982.

Chapter 15

MUTAGENIC ACTIVITY IN EXCREMENTS, SEWAGE, AND SLUDGE

Richard H. C. San

TABLE OF CONTENTS

I. INTRODUCTION

The introduction of mutagens and carcinogens into man's environment by industrial, agricultural, and other human activity has attracted considerable public concern and attention. Genotoxicity testing programs and regulatory decisions are focused on man-made chemicals such as pesticides, food additives, cosmetics, pharmaceutical products, as well as industrial emissions (air and water pollutants). Much less consideration has been given to mutagens released into the environment by natural processes.

Several studies have demonstrated the formation and presence of mutagens within the feces of mammals: nitrosamine production resulting from nitrosation,[1-3] formation of nitroso compounds due to transnitrosation controlled by bacterial enzymes,[4] production of mutagenic metabolites of bile through the activity of fecal bacteria,[5] and the presence of water-soluble mutagens.[6]

Human and animal excrements are commonly used as fertilizers in agriculture. The quantity of human and animal excreta produced on an annual basis is staggering. In the U.S. alone, the yearly production is estimated to be more than 2 billion tons. If these materials do contain genotoxic components which are stable over an extended period of time, the magnitude of environmental contamination by excrements is considerable.

This chapter concerns some of the studies conducted in our laboratory to assess whether fecal components constitute a substantial source of environmental mutagens.

II. FECAL MUTAGENS FROM CARNIVOROUS AND HERBIVOROUS ANIMALS

In an attempt to illustrate whether the presence of mutagens in feces is confined to certain animal species, Stich et al.[7] examined the fecal material from both carnivorous and herbivorous animals for genotoxic activity. Chloroform-methanol extracts from the feces of three carnivores (dog, river otter, and seagull) and five herbivores (cow, horse, sheep, chicken, and goose) all induced severe chromosome aberrations (breaks and exchanges) in cultured Chinese hamster ovary (CHO) cells. The data indicate variations in the potency of the fecal extracts among the species examined. Although an accurate comparison between different species was difficult, one obvious conclusion from the study was that genotoxic activity was demonstrable in the feces of both herbivorous and carnivorous animals.

III. STABILITY OF FECAL MUTAGENS IN THE ENVIRONMENT

The mere presence of genotoxic activity in animal excrements is inadequate evidence that such materials constitute a source of environmental mutagens. Unless these substances are stable, their contribution toward the total load of mutagens in the environment may be minimal.

Preliminary studies were conducted to determine the stability of the genotoxic material in cow and human feces sampled at different intervals after deposition.[8] The chromosome-damaging activity in cow and heifer feces did not change significantly following storage over a 7-week period at natural temperatures varying daily from 14 to 27°C. Human feces also retained their chromosome-breaking properties over a period of 7 weeks (Table 1). It remains to be shown whether the observed chromosome-damaging activity is due to (1) the persistence of clastogenic agents present in the freshly deposited species or (2) the formation of new genotoxic compounds. There is evidence that mutagens could be formed within excrement in vitro.[9]

IV. GENOTOXICITY OF HUMAN SEWAGE

In order to determine whether human fecal mutagens actually enter the environment, it is necessary to follow the distribution, dilution, and survival of the genotoxic activity in

Table 1
SURVIVAL OF CHROMOSOME-BREAKING ACTIVITY IN HUMAN AND ANIMAL EXCRETA FOLLOWING STORAGE AT "NATURAL" TEMPERATURES (14—27°C)

Weeks after excretion	Dilution of fecal extract	Chromosome aberrations[a]				
		Cow 1:10	Heifer 1:10	Human		
				1:10	1:20	1:40
0		34.8 (0.51)[b]	16.7(0.29)	M.I.[c]	M.I.	7.8(0.17)
2		36.8(0.50)	13.0(0.13)	M.I.	M.I.	13.4(0.23)
7		28.5(0.38)	10.3(0.13)	53.1(0.87)	7.6 (0.02)	4.6(0.05)

[a] Chinese hamster ovary cells were exposed to the fecal extract for 3 hr, arrested at metaphase with colchicine (for 4 hr) at 16 hr post-treatment.

[b] Chromosome aberrations are expressed as percentages of metaphase plates with at least one chromatid break or exchange. Numbers in parentheses show the average number of chromatid exchanges per metaphase plate. In control cultures without any exposure to fecal extracts, less than 1% of the metaphase spreads show chromatid/chromosome aberrations.

[c] M.I. = mitotic inhibition (less than one metaphase spread among 6000 cells).

Table 2
CHROMOSOME ABERRATIONS IN CHINESE HAMSTER OVARY CELLS FOLLOWING A 3-HR EXPOSURE TO EXTRACTS FROM WATER AND BOTTOM SEDIMENTS AT A SEWAGE OUTFALL

Dilution of extract	Percent metaphases with chromosome aberrations			
	At sewage outfall		Upstream from outfall	
	Site 1	Site 2	Site 1	Site 2
Bottom sediment				
1:15	25.6	30.2	3.0	1.6
1:20	17.9	19.1	0.8	1.0
Water sample				
1:10	44.7	11.0	3.6	3.3
1:12.5	12.4	4.2	0.8	0.0
1:15	3.2	3.1	0.8	2.6

sewage. One suitable candidate for such an investigation is the sewage-carrying creek in the residential areas of a community without any sewage treatment facility and industrial contamination.[10] Freeze-dried mud and water samples as well as concentrates prepared by solvent extraction procedures induced chromosome aberrations in CHO cells following a 3-hr exposure (Table 2). Water and mud collected upstream from the sewage outfall did not reveal any significant clastogenic activity (Table 2). Tests on samples from other sewage outfalls and upstream locations confirmed these observations.

Table 3
GENOTOXIC ACTIVITY IN
TREATED HUMAN SEWAGE
SLUDGE[a]

Dilution of extract	Percent metaphases with chromosome aberrations	
	Sample 1	Sample 2
1:10	M.I.[b]	T[b]
1:15	60.9	T
1:17.5	46.2	T
1:20	38.3	12.9
1:25	27.7	8.0
1:30	10.0	0
1:35	6.6	0
1:40	7.2	0
Control (no extract)	0	

[a] Commercially available as fertilizer. Extracts were tested for chromosome-damaging activity on Chinese hamster ovary cells. The two samples were from different suppliers.
[b] M.I. = mitotic inhibition; T = toxic.

V. TREATED HUMAN SEWAGE SLUDGE

In view of the large quantities of treated human sewage sludge being used as fertilizer, the possibility remains that such usage may constitute a source of environmental mutagens. Two commercially available samples were examined for chromosome-damaging activity in CHO cells.[11] The water-methanol extract from both samples induced chromosome aberrations in CHO cells (Table 3).

VI. ORGANIC FERTILIZERS PREPARED FROM ANIMAL EXCRETA

Commercially available chicken manure, steer manure, and materials from local stables (composted horse manure) are examples of organic fertilizers used in vegetable gardens. The water-methanol extract from these samples exhibited chromosome-damaging activity in CHO cells (Table 4).[12]

Another source of organic fertilizer is the slurry from cattle feed lots. The slurry is collected in an underground concrete holding tank, stored for up to 5 months, and then used as fertilizer. Water-methanol extracts from the slurry collected inside the feed lot as well as in the holding tank demonstrated strong chromosome-damaging activity in CHO cells (Table 5).[12]

VII. DISCUSSION

The magnitude of environmental contamination by fecal mutagens remains to be determined. Considering the large quantities of animal and human wastes produced daily, the amount of mutagens released into the environment is by no means insignificant. The following numbers provide an idea of the amount of excrement produced per day: cattle, 38 to 74 lb (wet weight); hogs, 2.8 to 9.5 lb; dogs, about 0.3 lb; chickens, 0.1 to 0.4 lb; turkeys, 1 lb; man, about 0.4 lb.[13,14] In 1970 in the U.S., there were about 91 million beef cattle, 15

Table 4
GENOTOXIC ACTIVITY IN ORGANIC FERTILIZERS
PREPARED FROM ANIMAL EXCRETA

Dilution of extract	Percent metaphases with chromosome aberrations		
	Chicken manure[a]	Steer manure[a]	Composted horse manure
1:3.3	—[b]	—	M.I.[b]
1:5	T[b]	T	25.0
1:6	M.I.	M.I.	—
1:7	17.3	19.1	—
1:8	3.6	2.7	6.0
1:10	0.9	0	0

Note: All extracts were tested for chromosome-damaging activity on Chinese hamster ovary cells.

[a] Commercially available as fertilizer.
[b] "—" = not tested; T = toxic; M.I. = mitotic inhibition.

Table 5
CHROMOSOME ABERRATIONS IN CHINESE
HAMSTER OVARY CELLS FOLLOWING A 3-HR
EXPOSURE TO EXTRACT OF SLURRY FROM
CALF FEED LOT

Dilution of extract	Metabolic activation	Percent metaphases with chromosome aberrations	
		−	+[a]
1:8		40.0	T[b]
1:10		26.1	T
1:12.5		12.4	M.I.[b]
1:15		13.0	77.7
1:17.5		6.0	64.5
1:20		0	32.7
1:25		0	16.1
1:30		0	5.9
1:35		0	3.9

[a] Test conducted in the presence of an Aroclor 1254-induced rat liver homogenate to provide metabolic activation system.
[b] T = toxic; M.I. = mitotic inhibition.

million dairy cattle, 57 million swine, 4 million broilers, 6 million horses, 27 million dogs, and 220 million human beings. The annual total of animal and human wastes amounts to more than 2 billion tons. In the U.S. alone, the daily production of dog feces amounts to about 3500 tons.[15]

In connection with environmental pollution, the effectiveness of sewage treatment in the removal of fecal mutagens warrants some consideration. The sewage is subjected to bacterial degradation in lagoons or, in primary or secondary treatment plants, allowed to sediment in tanks prior to anaerobic digestion with bacteria. In all three procedures, the liquid phase is discharged periodically into receiving waters. The sludge is transferred to landfill sites, burnt or recycled for use as fertilizer. Present sewage treatment procedures are designed to eliminate microorganisms and parasites. The removal of chemical contaminants, let alone genotoxic agents, is not the major consideration. Current studies indicate the presence of genotoxic material in treated sewage,[16] in municipal sewage landfill sites,[17] and in sewage sludge processed for use as fertilizer.[11] This raises questions about the penetration of genotoxic agents into soil, their presence in runoff water, their uptake by plants, and possible re-entry into the human food chain.

Another area of concern is the proposed recycling of treated sewage sludge as supplementary cattle feed. Experiments indicate that treated sludge has half the nutritive value of cottonseed meal.[18] Until the development of acceptable methods for removal of microorganisms and chemical contaminants, the recycling of sludge as cattle feed may provide a convenient means for the distribution of fecal mutagens.

Information on the distribution, dilution, and survival of the genotoxic agents in sewage, sludge, and cattle feed lots are prerequisites to properly assess whether these materials present a potential or actual health hazard to man as well as to animals and plants.

REFERENCES

1. **Bruce, W. R., Varghese, A. J., Furrer, R., and Land, P. C.,** A mutagen in the feces of normal humans, in *Origins of Human Cancer,* Hiatt, H. H., Watson, J. D., and Winsten, J. A., Eds., Cold Spring Harbor Laboratory, Cold Spring Harbor, N.Y., 1977, 1641.
2. **Varghese, A. J., Land, P. C., Furrer, R., and Bruce, W. R.,** Non-volatile N-nitroso compounds in human feces, in *Environmental Aspects of N-Nitroso Compounds,* Walker, E. A., Castegnaro, M., Griciute, L., and Lyle, R. E., Eds., IARC Sci. Publ. No. 19, International Agency for Research on Cancer, Lyon, France, 1978, 257.
3. **Wang, T., Kakizoe, T., Dion, P., Furrer, R., Varghese, A. J., and Bruce, W. R.,** Volatile nitrosamines in normal human feces, *Nature (London), 276,* 280, 1978.
4. **Mandel, M., Ichinotsubo, D., and Mower, H.,** Nitroso group exchange as a way of activation of nitrosamines by bacteria, *Nature (London), 267,* 248, 1977.
5. **Karpinsky, G. E., McCoy, E. C., and Rosenkranz, H. S.,** Conversion of human bile to mutagens by human-derived strains of *Bacteriodes fragilis, 10th Annu. Meet. Environ. Mutagen Soc. U.S.,* Abstr., 62, 1979.
6. **Stich, H. F. and Kuhnlein, U.,** Chromosome breaking activity of human feces and its enhancement by transition metals, *Int. J. Cancer, 24,* 284, 1979.
7. **Stich, H. F., Stich, W., and Acton, A. B.,** Mutagenicity of fecal extracts from carnivorous and herbivorous animals, *Mutat. Res., 78,* 105, 1980.
8. **San, R. H. C., Stich, H. F., and Acton, A. B.,** Persistence of chromosome and DNA damaging activity and DNA repair inhibiting action of human and animal excreta (Abstract), *11th Annu. Meet. Environ. Mutagen Soc. U.S.,* Nashville, Tenn., March 16-20, 1980.
9. **Macdonald, I. A. and Rao, B. G.,** Nitrite-induced fecal mutagens: some preliminary studies, *Cancer, 49,* 1405, 1982.
10. **San, R. H. C., Stich, H. F., Acton, A. B., and Maus, L.,** Human sewage: a source of environmental mutagens? *Environ. Mutagenesis, 3,* 350, 1981.
11. **San, R. H. C. and Acton, A. B.,** Genotoxicity of organic fertilizers: treated human sewage sludge, slurry from cattle feed lot and chicken manure, manuscript in preparation, 1982.
12. **San, R. H. C.,** unpublished data, 1982.
13. **Loehr, R. C.,** Animal wastes, a national problem, *J. Sanitation Eng. Div. Am. Soc. Civ. Eng., 95,* 189, 1969.
14. **Taiganides, E. P. and Hazen, T. E.,** Properties of farm animal excreta, *Trans. ASAE, 9,* 374, 1966.
15. **Djerassi, C., Israel, A., and Jochle, W.,** Planned parenthood for pets? *Bull. Atom. Sci., 29,* 10, 1973.
16. **Saxema, J. and Schwartz, D. J.,** Mutagens in wastewaters renovated by advanced wastewater treatment, *Bull. Environ. Contaminants Toxicol., 22,* 319, 1979.
17. **Plewa, M. J., Wagner, E. D., Wood, S., and Hopke, P. K.,** Mutagenicity of Chicago sewage sludge in *Zea mays* and *Tradescantia paludosa* (Abstract), *12th Annu. Meet. Environ. Mutagen Soc. U.S.,* San Diego, Calif, March 5—8, 1981.
18. **Krishnamurthy, S. K.,** Reusing the city's sewage — radiation could be the answer, *Nucl. India, 17,* 1, 1979.

Chapter 16

MUTAGENICITY OF MUNICIPAL SEWAGE SLUDGE

Michael J. Plewa and Philip K. Hopke

TABLE OF CONTENTS

I. INTRODUCTION

A major problem facing the U.S. is the disposal of the sludge resulting from the treatment of municipal sewage. There has been a substantial increase in the number and efficiency of sewage treatment plants in the past decade particularly in suburban and rural areas, resulting in an increased amount of sludge requiring disposal. In addition, previously employed sludge disposal methods such as ocean dumping are soon to be severely limited or stopped entirely. The incineration of sludge requires expensive facilities and may result in increased air pollution. An attractive alternative disposal method is the application of this organic matter to agricultural lands or its use in the reclamation of land stripped of its organic matter by surface mining.

However, there may be problems associated with sludge disposal by land application. Analyses of sludge from the Calumet and Southwest treatment plants of the Metropolitan Sanitary District of Chicago, indicated that concentrations of several heavy metals were substantially higher than in typical soil compositions. Thus, in 1967, a large demonstration and research program was initiated to examine the feasibility of land application of digested sewage sludge from the Metropolitan Sanitary District of Chicago wastewater treatment plants. A major objective was to examine compositional changes in soil, crops, and water from sludge-amended fields.

In the intervening period, there has been a great deal of study on the uptake and accumulation of heavy metals (most notably zinc and cadmium) in corn *(Zea mays)*, the effects of these elements on soil bacteria, and the potential for transmission of heavy metals through a food chain that might result in impact on the public health.[1-6] It has been found that zinc and cadmium accumulate in corn grain and leaf tissues.[5,6] High levels of sludge treatment appear to inhibit the development of several inbred strains of corn but do not cause overt symptoms of metal toxicity.[6] Studies of the long-term effects of sludge in the food chain and on field productivity are in progress.

Additional contaminants that may be present in municipal sewage sludge are naturally occurring organic compounds and compounds from industrial processes or other anthropogenic activities. One of the particular concerns related to these organic compounds is the possibility of mutagenic compounds being released into the environment. The lack of understanding of the distribution and fate of mutagens present in sewage sludge and their long-term effects following land application requires additional study. An environmental mutagen or genotoxin is an agent that is released into the environment that can alter the genetic material or alter the proper functioning of the genetic material. The presence of such genotoxic agents in the environment is a serious threat to the public health.[7-9] Depending upon the developmental stage of an individual a genotoxin can exert teratogenic effects,[7,10,11] precipitate coronary disease,[12] produce mutations involving germinal cells,[8,10,13] or cause mutations in somatic cells that may become neoplastic.[7,8,14-16]

It is widely believed by scientists that the majority of human cancers are due to the presence of chemical carcinogens in the environment.[14,16,17] The somatic cell mutation theory of cancer revolves around the simple premise that cancer arises in humans and other organisms through damage to DNA, to chromosomes, or to mitotic recombination.[16] During the last decade evidence has been reported which demonstrates that most, if not all, chemical carcinogens are mutagens.[7,16-19] Research conducted in the U.S., Japan, and the U.K. demonstrated a high correlation between carcinogenicity and mutagenicity in *Salmonella* (r = 0.85 to 0.93), indicating that environmental mutagens play a significant role in the induction of human cancer.[20-23]

Besides the induction of somatic cell mutations, environmental mutagens induce mutations in a second tissue type. Genetic damage by environmental mutagens to germinal cells has by far the most serious consequences when one considers adverse long-term effects upon our species. With somatic cell damage an effect is realized usually within a single generation and the death of an individual is the most serious consequence. However, the induction of germ cell mutational damage transcends the usual generational boundary of toxicology. Now we face a situation in which not only an exposed person has the possibility of deleterious effects but also his progeny, generation upon generation. The probability that environmental mutagens will increase the genetic load of our species through an increased mutation rate in germinal cells is the greatest danger posed by these genotoxic agents. In a metropolitan area such as Chicago there are major chemical, petrochemical, petroleum-refining, and other industries that utilize organic chemicals in large quantities. Other activities such as fossil fuel combustion produce genotoxic compounds that may enter the sanitary sewer system. Therefore, there exists the possibility that genotoxic compounds present in sewage sludge may be released into the environment by leaching into surface or ground water or may be incorporated into the human food chain through the use of sewage sludge as a soil additive.

The type of wastewater treatment process influences the quantities of sludge produced. Harrington[24] suggested an estimate of sludge production of 0.113 kg per capita per day of suspended solids in sewage. Each year the approximately 162 million people served by municipal sewage treatment facilities in the U.S. generate 4.5 to 5.4 million dry metric tons of sludge. Advanced treatment of sewage would increase the quantity of dry solids to approximately 0.159 kg per capita per day. If secondary treatment of sewage were conducted at all existing sewage treatment plants the annual quantity of sludge would be approximately 9 million dry metric tons.

II. METHODS IN ANALYZING THE MUTAGENIC POTENTIAL OF SEWAGE SLUDGES

The primary approaches that have been applied in the evaluation of the mutagenicity of sewage sludges include *in situ* monitoring, in vivo laboratory assays of whole sludges, and fractionation plus assay methods.

A. *In Situ* Monitoring

When sewage sludge is disposed by soil amendment, the fields themselves may be monitored for the presence of mutagens by measuring the induction of mutation in plants of specific genotypes.

An *in situ* study of the possible mutagenic effects of municipal sewage sludge was conducted between May and August 1979. The experiment incorporated multiple genetic end points to analyze sludge from the Calumet and Southwest sewage facilities of the Metropolitan Sanitary District of Chicago. Test plots were constructed on the NW900 plots at the University of Illinois Agronomy Research Center near Elwood. A history of these plots covering the period 1968 to 1979 was compiled and it was determined that the plots were suitable. If *in situ* studies are to be valid, it is important to know the past history of such plots since prior application of mutagenic substances could seriously interfere with the planned studies. It is particularly important to know that the sample and control areas have the same history so that the controls properly reflect the base conditions of the study. The NW900 test plot had four levels of sludge application in 1979. The control plot received no sludge application and adequate nitrogen was provided by soil application of chemical fertilizer. The maximum treatment plot received 17.8 cm of liquid sludge which was equivalent to approximately 21.0 Tg/ha of dry material. Two other treatment plots received one half and one fourth of the amount of sludge delivered to the maximum treatment plot. No pesticides were applied to any of the test plots.

The genetic end point was reverse mutation at the *waxy (wx)* locus of pollen grains in *Zea mays* (maize) plants. The *wx* locus is located on chromosome 9 of *Z. mays* at map position 9—59.[25] The *wx* locus controls the synthesis of the starch amylose. When used in this assay, pollen grains (microgametophytes) operate as functional haploids and express their genetic constitution rather than that of their parental sporophyte. A pollen grain that carries a dominant allele (*Wx*) can synthesize amylose as part of its starch component. Amylose, when reacted with iodine, turns a dark blue-black color[26] and *Wx* grains will therefore stain blue-black. A pollen grain that carries the recessive allele *(wx)* cannot synthesize amylose and will appear tan when reacted with iodine. Thus, the color of the pollen grain after staining with iodine gives a clear indication of its genotype. Genetic reversion of *wx* to *Wx* can be quantitatively determined by counting the number of black stained pollen grains within the field of tan stained grains. In the forward mutation assay, *Wx* to *wx*, tan stained forward mutant grains are counted in a field of black stained pollen grains. In each case the frequency of mutant pollen grains is determined by counting individual mutant grains and estimating the number of viable pollen grains by counting the number present in 20 randomly selected 1 mm^2 areas and multiplying by the slide area. The maize *wx* locus assay has been used for *in situ* and laboratory studies on mutagenesis.[27-29]

In the tests on sewage sludge, *Z. mays* kernels of inbred M14 homozygous for either the *wx-C* or the *wx-90* heteroallele were used. One row of each heteroallele type was planted in a control plot and in each of three treatment plots. The plants grew until early anthesis when each tassel was individually labeled, harvested, and stored in 70% ethanol for subsequent analysis. Pollen grains were removed from the tassels and analyzed as described by Plewa and Wagner.[29] The frequency of revertant pollen grains was determined by dividing the total number of revertant grains by the total number of viable pollen grains. The percentage of clear, collapsed, aborted pollen grains was also determined by estimating the number of aborted pollen grains and dividing by the sum of the viable plus the aborted grains.

The data for the induction of revertant pollen grains at the *wx-C* and *wx-90* heteroalleles from *Z. mays* grown in the sludge test plots are presented in Table 1. For the *wx-C* allele, over 5 million pollen grains were analyzed. The frequency of reverse mutation did not increase with the increased amount of sewage sludge added to the soil. However, a direct relationship was observed between the amount of applied sludge and the frequency of pollen abortions within the range of 19.4% for the control to 49.9% in the highest treatment group. The relationship between the abortion frequency in plants homozygous for *wx-C* and concentration of amended sludge indicated an increased rate of gametophytic death. Thus, for this heteroallele, some agent in the sludge was toxic to the developing pollen grains. No increased frequency of revertants in the *wx-C* heteroallele was seen and may be due in part to the observed toxicity.

A different result was obtained for the *wx-90* reversion tests. In an experiment that involved the analysis of over 5 million pollen grains there was an increased frequency of revertants with increased sludge amendment for the half-maximum and maximum treatment plots. In the control plots, the frequency of revertants was 1.6×10^{-6}; plants grown in the half-maximum sludge plots exhibited a reversion frequency that was twice that of the controls. There was a 10-fold increase in the frequency of revertants for the highest treatment group. The percentage of pollen abortion was constant among the control and treatment groups. The sludge apparently was not toxic to the developing pollen grains with this genotype.

These data indicate that these two heteroalleles express different responses to components that are present in sludge. Although the molecular nature of the lesions in the *wx-C* and *wx-90* heteroalleles are not known, it has been suggested that *wx-C* is a base-pair substitution.[30] A difference in the specific types of lesions may account for the differences in response to sludge exposure.

1. Other Possible In Situ Genetic Monitors

Several other higher plant systems are available as monitors of environmental mutagens that could be employed *in situ* in the evaluation of sewage sludges. Such assays include the

Table 1

SUMMARY OF DATA FOR *wx* REVERSION IN THE *IN SITU* TESTS

Experiment no.	No. mutant pollen grains	No. viable pollen grains	Abortion (%)	Frequency of mutant pollen grains
wx-C inbred M14				
4336-C	37	1,267,963	19.4	2.9×10^{-5}
4338	17	1,052,855	36.5	1.6×10^{-5}
4340	5	1,429,642	46.5	3.5×10^{-6}
4342	6	1,299,568	49.9	4.6×10^{-6}
wx-90 inbred M14				
4335-C	2	1,266,242	27.9	1.6×10^{-6}
4337	2	1,268,930	26.6	1.6×10^{-6}
4339	4	1,256,245	29.9	3.2×10^{-6}
4341	22	1,212,922	28.2	1.8×10^{-5}

wx locus assay in barley,[31] the chlorophyll-deficient mutation assay in barley,[32] the *yellow-green-2* locus assay in maize,[33,34] the *alcohol dehydrogenase-1* locus assay in maize,[35-37] somatic crossing over in soybean,[38,39] and the use of micronucleus induction in tetrads or mutation induction in stamen hairs of *Tradescantia*.[40-42] The advantages of using plant systems for *in situ* assays include:

1.   A number of well defined genetic assays are available.
2.   Plants usually have a sufficiently long period of sensitivity so that chronic exposure data may be obtained.
3.   Plant systems are usually easy to maintain and are inexpensive.

2. The Requirements for In Situ Genetic Assays

Adequate *in situ* monitoring for environmental mutagens must meet seven basic requirements:

1.   A knowledge of the history of the area to be assayed.
2.   The construction of test plots with proper controls.
3.   The use of well defined assays with discrete and calibrated genetic end points.
4.   The use of appropriate numbers of indicator organisms to provide a sufficiently large data base for each test plot.
5.   Trained personnel to maintain the test plots and to label and harvest the plants at the appropriate time.
6.   Laboratory personnel to conduct the careful and competent analysis of the expressed phenotype and the proper interpretation of the measured genetic events.
7.   The use of appropriate statistical methods in the evaluation of the data.

B. In Vivo Laboratory Assays of Whole Sludge

A second approach to assay the mutagenic properties of whole or concentrated whole sewage sludge involves the use of plant genetic indicator organisms exposed to samples of sludge under laboratory conditions. The use of intact organisms under laboratory conditions provides for the verification of positive responses from *in situ* studies. The fact that the same unmodified sludge may be studied *in situ* and in the laboratory makes this approach relevant to realistic environmental situations.

Whole sludge and concentrated whole sludge samples obtained from various treatment facilities in Illinois have been evaluated for their potential to induce forward mutation in *Zea mays* and micronucleic in *Tradescantia paludosa*.

1. Studies with Early-Early Synthetic Zea mays

An experiment for assaying whole sludge with a specially designed maize inbred was conducted by Hopke et al.[43] Early-Early Synthetic is a rapidly maturing inbred and develops from kernel to tassel emergence in approximately 4 weeks. The inbred reaches a height of approximately 50 cm and can be grown in 10-cm diameter pots. With these convenient growth characteristics Early-Early Synthetic can be used in plant growth chambers where well-controlled conditions can be assured. Also higher concentrations of sludge could be administered to the plants than in the *in situ* study. Five plants were grown as a control group in individual 10-cm diameter plastic pots filled with a standard soil mixture and watered with deionized water. Standard potting soil consisted of four parts loam, two parts peat moss, and one part sand. The plants were given adequate chemical fertilizer. Three treatment groups of five plants each were exposed to different amounts of sludge added to the initial soil mixture. For the highest treatment group, one part sludge was added to two parts of standard soil. These plants were watered with a 1/3 dilution of sludge in deionized water. For the intermediate treatment group, one part sludge was added to five parts of soil. The plants were watered with a 1/6 dilution of sludge. In the lowest treatment group, 11 parts of soil were combined with one part of sludge and these plants were watered with a 1/12 sludge/deionized water solution. Plants were grown in a plant growth chamber adjusted to a 17-hr photoperiod of 300 μEinsteins/m^2/sec with day and night temperatures of 25 and 20°C, respectively. The plants in the treatment groups were watered with the appropriately diluted sludge until tassel emergence and then watered with deionized water only. At early anthesis the tassels were harvested, labeled, and stored in 70% ethanol for subsequent analysis. The pollen grains were analyzed for forward mutants.

The plants used in this test were homozygous for the dominant *Wx* allele. Forward mutation to a recessive *wx* allele causes the mutant pollen grain to stain tan after treatment with an iodine stain. A forward mutation test detects a broader range of mutational events than a reverse mutation test.

The results of the induction of forward mutation at the *wx* locus in Early-Early Synthetic maize by the Chicago sludge sample are presented in Table 2. The data clearly show that the administration of Chicago sludge increased the frequency of mutation by two orders of magnitude. The control frequency of mutant pollen grains of 4.3×10^{-5} is consistent with spontaneous frequencies observed in other studies with this inbred.[29] The frequencies of mutant pollen grains decreased with increasing amounts of added sludge indicating that even the lowest concentration of applied Chicago sludge is high enough to reach the toxic region of the mutational dose-response curve. The percentage of pollen abortions is higher at the higher sludge concentrations than the control group. The control frequency is 13.3% while it is 19.9% in the highest treatment group. There is, however, no dose-dependence to the abortion data. There is a clear indication that Chicago sludge induced forward mutation in the pollen grains with a substantial increase in frequency over the control group value. The increased abortion rate indicated the presence of toxic as well as mutagenic agents.

A similar experiment was conducted using sludge obtained from the Champaign, Illinois wastewater treatment plant. Within the statistical limits of the experiment, the sludge sample did not induce an increased frequency of forward mutations in this assay.

2. Studies on the Induction of Micronuclei in Tradescantia

The *Tradescantia paludosa* micronucleus test detects chromosome damage in tetrads following meiosis of the pollen grain mother cells.[41] A micronucleus may result from the induction of a multipolar nuclear division or by chromosome aberrations that result in acentric fragments. The fragment of broken chromosome can be observed as a separate micronucleus within the tetrad.

Inflorescences of *Tradescantia* from clone 03 plants were obtained from T. H. Ma (Western Illinois University, Macomb). The use of a single clone ensured that all of the inflorescences

Table 2
FORWARD MUTATION AT THE MAIZE *wx* LOCUS INDUCED BY
CHICAGO SEWAGE SLUDGE

Treatment	No. of mutants	No. of pollen grains analyzed	Frequency mutant pollen grains	Pollen abortion (%)	Statistic
Control	34	788,000	4.3×10^{-5}	13.3	
Low (1/12) concentration	7,585	825,000	9.2×10^{-3}	17.1	$p < 0.001$
Medium (1/6) concentration	5,650	898,000	6.4×10^{-3}	20.4	$p < 0.001$
High (1/3) concentration	1,776	836,000	2.1×10^{-3}	19.9	$p < 0.001$

were isogenic. The plants were vegetatively propagated and grown under greenhouse conditions. Inflorescences were cut with stems approximately 3 to 4 cm in length. Typically 8 to 10 inflorescences were used for each treatment group. The cuttings were placed in test tubes containing various mixtures of sludge and Hoagland's solution.[44] A negative control of Hoagland's solution (a plant nutrient solution) and a positive control of 50 m*M* maleic hydrazide in Hoagland's solution were used for each experiment. The inflorescences were treated for 24 hr with the text mixture and then placed into Hoagland's solution only for an additional 24 hr. The solutions were aerated by bubbling water-saturated air through each tube. The temperature was maintained at 24°C using a water bath. After the treatment period, the inflorescences were removed from the treatment tubes and fixed in a solution of ethanol:glacial acetic acid (3:1, v:v) for 48 hr. The samples were then stored in 70% ethanol for subsequent analysis.

The analysis procedure for scoring the micronuclei-containing tetrads has been described by Ma.[41,42] The number of multiple micronuclei per tetrad was also recorded. The frequency of micronuclei induction was determined by dividing the total number of micronuclei observed by the number of tetrads analyzed. This ratio was multiplied by 100 to yield the number of micronuclei per 100 tetrads.

Samples of whole sludge and sludge concentrated by the removal of water were obtained from the Illinois cities of Chicago, Champaign, Hinsdale, and Kankakee.

a. Chicago Sludge

The results of the micronucleus test on whole Chicago sludge and various dilutions are presented in Table 3. The data clearly demonstrate a dose-dependent increase in the frequency of micronuclei with increased sludge concentration. Dilutions above 1/4 induced a significant increase in the frequency of micronuclei. Whole sludge, the 1/2 dilution, and the positive control induced an increased frequency of tetrads containing multiple micronuclei. Thus, whole Chicago sewage sludge and dilutions above 1/4 can induce cytogenetic damage in meiotic cells including multiple events in single tetrads.

An aqueous phase of Chicago sludge was prepared by removing the water from 10 ℓ of the sludge aqueous fraction by vacuum distillation and lyophilization. The resulting dry material was redissolved in 200 mℓ of distilled water. This solution was a 50X concentration of the original sludge aqueous fraction. Sterilized and nonsterilized Chicago sludge aqueous phase as well as 5X, 12.5X, and 25X concentrations were analyzed with *Tradescantia*. The data are presented in Table 4. A dose-dependent increase in the frequency of micronuclei was observed with the increase in the concentration factor of the Chicago sludge aqueous fraction. The unconcentrated or the 5X concentrated aqueous phase sample did not induce a significant increase in the frequency of micronuclei.

Table 3
INDUCTION OF MICRONUCLEI IN *TRADESCANTIA* BY CHICAGO MUNICIPAL SEWAGE SLUDGE

Treatment	No. of tetrads analyzed	Total no. micronuclei	Micronuclei/ 100 tetrads	Frequency of multiple micronuclei ($\times 10^{-3}$)
Experiment 1				
Control	9,980	337	3.4	2.7
1/16 dilution	4,654	160	3.7	3.2
1/8 dilution	4,958	185	3.7	1.8
1/4 dilution	6,471	234	3.6	2.2
1/2 dilution	5,691	273	4.8	4.7
Experiment 2				
Control	6,673	236	3.5	2.8
50 m*M* maleic hydrazide	3,176	358	11.3	6.0
Whole sludge	2,355	199	8.5	4.2
Experiment 3				
Control	8,056	294	3.6	3.6
50 m*M* maleic hydrazide	1,906	226	11.8	4.7
1/4 dilution	5,655	206	3.6	1.4
1/2 dilution	7,011	405	5.8	4.0
Whole sludge	10,627	889	8.4	7.8
Experiment 4				
Control	10,452	336	3.2	0.9
50 m*M* maleic hydrazide	4,517	425	9.4	9.1
1/4 dilution	8,656	301	3.5	2.5
1/2 dilution	5,955	290	4.9	2.9
Whole sludge	2,596	255	9.8	10.0

A series of tests was conducted on the acetone fraction of Chicago sewage sludge. The fraction was prepared by vacuum distilling an acetone extract of solid sludge material. The residue was redissolved in 0.5 mℓ dimethyl sulfoxide (DMSO). The DMSO solution was mixed with 9.5 mℓ of Hoagland's solution and assayed. No induction of micronuclei was detected with the acetone fraction (Table 4).

The *Tradescantia* tests with Chicago sludge indicate that agents are present that can inflict cytogenetic damage in meiotic cells of a higher eukaryote. It is interesting to note that the aqueous fraction is much less mutagenic than whole sludge and that the acetone fraction did not induce micronuclei.

b. Champaign Sludge

Whole sludge samples and a 1/2 dilution in Hoagland's solution were assayed for their ability to induce micronuclei. Neither of these samples induced a significant increase in cytogenetic damage (Table 5).

Whole sludge was concentrated by lyophilization. The solid sludge was then mixed with Hoagland's solution at proportions of 0.3 g:4.7 mℓ and 0.6 g:4.7 mℓ which corresponded to approximately 2X and 4X concentrations, respectively. The results of these experiments are presented in Table 6; none of the Champaign sludge samples induced a significant increase in the frequency of micronuclei.

c. Hinsdale Sludge

Whole sludge samples were assayed and a negative response was observed (Table 5). The Hinsdale sludge was concentrated by lyophilization. The sludge solids were mixed with

Table 4
RESULTS OF THE CHICAGO SLUDGE AQUEOUS
FRACTIONS AND ACETONE EXTRACTS WITH
THE *TRADESCANTIA* MICRONUCLEUS TEST

Treatment	No. tetrads	No. MCN	MCN/100 tetrads
Control	10,750	340	3.2 ± 0.50
Aqueous phase (nonsterilized)	23,514	813	3.5 ± 0.30
Aqueous phase (sterilized)	27,347	1,014	3.7 ± 0.50
Aqueous phase (25×)	7,531	664	8.8 ± 2.40
Acetone fraction	13,013	705	5.4 ± 1.10
Control	35,440	1,264	3.6 ± 0.51
Aqueous phase (5×)	15,300	760	5.0 ± 0.77
Aqueous phase (12.5×)	12,298	952	7.7 ± 1.50
Aqueous phase (25×)	8,175	866	10.6 ± 0.84
Acetone fraction	23,050	927	4.0 ± 0.43

Table 5
RESULTS OF DIFFERENT WHOLE SLUDGE SAMPLES
FROM FOUR CITIES WITH THE *TRADESCANTIA*
MICRONUCLEUS TEST

Sample	No. tetrads	No. MCN	MCN/100 tetrads
Control	6,174	180	2.92 ± 0.55
+ Control (50 m*M* MH)	8,887	972	10.94 ± 1.42
Chicago sludge	8,071	515	6.38 ± 1.61
Kankakee sludge	7,048	347	4.92 ± 0.80
Hinsdale sludge	6,333	314	4.48 ± 0.74
Champaign sludge (Sample 1)	8,225	342	4.16 ± 0.57
Champaign sludge (Sample 2)	6,460	282	4.37 ± 0.57

Hoagland's solution at proportions of 1 g:5 mℓ, 2 g:5 mℓ, and 3 g:5 mℓ which corresponded to 6.7X, 13.3X, and 20.0X concentrations, respectively. The data for the concentrated Hinsdale sludge are presented in Table 6. The concentrated Hinsdale sludge samples did not significantly increase the induction of micronuclei. These data agree with the results obtained with whole Hinsdale sludge.

d. Kankakee Sludge

Kankakee whole sludge samples were assayed and found to be negative (Table 5). Whole sludge was concentrated by lyophilization and 6.7X, 13.3X, and 20.0X concentrations in Hoagland's solution were prepared and assayed. The results are presented in Table 6 and only the 20X sludge concentration induced a positive response. Thus, it appears that a low concentration of mutagen(s) is present in Kankakee sludge that can induce chromosome damage in meiotic cells of *Tradescantia*.

Table 6
RESULTS OF CONCENTRATED SLUDGE SAMPLES
FROM SEVERAL CITIES WITH THE *TRADESCANTIA*
MICRONUCLEUS TEST

Sample	No. tetrads	No. MCN	MCN/100 tetrads
Control	5,297	200	3.8 ± 0.60
+ Control (50 m*M* MH)	7,989	445	5.6 ± 1.35
Kankakee sludge (6.7×)	5,486	348	6.3 ± 0.88
Kankakee sludge (13.3×)	6,408	404	6.3 ± 0.76
Kankakee sludge (20.0×)	3,027	298	9.8 ± 2.71
Control	10,449	539	5.2 ± 0.63
+ Control (50 m*M* MH)	15,032	1,263	8.4 ± 1.57
Hinsdale sludge (6.7×)	10,030	610	6.1 ± 0.86
Hinsdale sludge (13.3×)	6,271	319	5.1 ± 1.00
Hinsdale sludge (20.0×)	7,202	447	6.2 ± 1.10
Champaign sludge (2×)	10,263	460	4.5 ± 0.57
Champaign sludge (4×)	10,051	533	5.3 ± 1.03

3. Other Potential Genetic Assays for the Analysis of Whole Sludge or Sludge Concentrates

Additional genetic assays could be incorporated in an evaluation of whole or concentrated whole sludges. Since plants can grow in sludge/soil mixtures for extended time periods the same assays that were suggested for *in situ* use would be amenable to laboratory analysis. The soybean assay for mitotic segregation[38,39] and the yg-2 locus test in maize[33,34] are especially attractive.

C. Fractionation Plus Assay Methods

Various chemical extraction methodologies separate and concentrate organic compounds for subsequent analysis with short-term genetic tests. Combining these fractionation techniques with short-term tests provides for the detection and isolation of specific mutagenic agents from complex environmental mixtures. An excellent review on the use of short-term genetic assays in the isolation and identification of mutagens in complex mixtures has been published by Epler.[45] Complex mixtures such as tobacco smoke condensates,[46-48] plant products,[49-52] food,[51,52] hair dyes,[53] soots,[54] fly ash,[55] particulates from urban air,[56-59] petroleum products,[45] urine,[60] feces,[61] and sewage sludges,[43] have been evaluated for their mutagenic properties by fractionation plus assay methods. Epler[45] has identified four extraction methods used in the analysis of complex mixtures. These are (1) organic extraction, (2) aqueous extraction, (3) resin concentration and extraction, and (4) fractionation by chemical classes.

We have fractionated four municipal sewage sludges and have analyzed each subsequent fraction for mutagenicity in strains TA98 and TA100 of *Salmonella typhimurium*. The initial studies were conducted on a sample of Chicago sewage sludge from the Southwest Treatment Plant of the Chicago Municipal Sanitary District at Stickney, Illinois. This sample was obtained from the storage tanks of the University of Illinois Agronomy Research Center at

Elwood where it was stored before being applied to the fields. This sample was a composite of the sludge received at Elwood during the period from November 1978 to July 1979. The fractionation was conducted as follows. Sixteen liters (16 ℓ) of sewage sludge were centrifuged at 12,500 r/min in a Sorvall GSA rotor (max 25400 xg) for 60 min. One liter (1 ℓ) of the supernatant liquid was filter-sterilized by passing through a 0.45 μm Millipore filter (fraction A1). Another 2 ℓ of supernatant liquid were passed through a column of XAD-2 resin previously cleaned as recommended by Junk et al.[62] The column was eluted with 200 mℓ of methanol (fraction A2a), and then with 200 mℓ of diethylether (fraction A2b); 2 mℓ of dimethyl sulfoxide (DMSO) were added to each eluate. The eluates were reduced in volume on a rotoevaporator until only the DMSO solution remained. In addition, 10 ℓ of supernatant were concentrated 100-fold by vacuum distillation at 30°C (fraction A3). Each of these samples was tested for mutagenicity in the TA98 and TA100 strains with and without mammalian microsomal activation except for fraction A3. Fraction A3 was highly contaminated with bacteria and could not be filter sterilized because of its high viscosity.

The 2.5 kg solid pellet was extracted three times with 2 vol of acetone and the extracts were pooled (fraction E1). The residue was extracted three times with 1 vol of n-hexane and these extracts were pooled (fraction E2); 15 mℓ of DMSO were added to both the acetone and hexane extracts and each extract was concentrated. It was necessary to lyophilize fraction E1 to remove the residual water sequestered from the solid by the acetone. These solutions were filter sterilized and assayed for mutagenicity.

To determine the amount of mutagenic activity recovered by the acetone extraction, another 100 g of pellet obtained from a different subsample of sludge were extracted three times with 200 mℓ of acetone. The extracts were tested separately as fractions F1, F2, and F3. The weight of material dissolved in each fraction was measured by evaporation of 200 μℓ and 500 μℓ aliquots to dryness in a desiccator. The residue remaining was weighed and the concentration of acetone-soluble material in each fraction was calculated. Fifty milliliters (50 mℓ) of each fraction were dried over anhydrous sodium sulfate; 5 mℓ of DMSO were added and each fraction was concentrated as previously described.

Additional single grab samples were obtained from municipal treatment plants in Champaign (CHMP), Hinsdale (HNSD), Kankakee (KANK), and Sauget (SAUG). The Chicago (CHI) sample described above was also studied further.

The protocol for extracting the sludge was altered in order that the crude extracts could be fractionated in better defined chemical classes. This protocol is outlined in Figure 1. Chloroform:methanol was chosen because it is considerably less polar than acetone. This modification had advantages in that it permitted further chemical fractionation of the crude extracts and it reduced the amount of water sequestered during the extraction of the wet solids. The sequestered water was eliminated by extracting lyophilized solids rather than wet solids.

The crude extracts were then subjected to a further fractionation as outlined in Figure 2. These additional separation steps were necessary to determine the presence of mutagenic activity and to minimize synergistic and antagonistic effects of other species potentially present in these complex mixtures. This procedure separated the extracts into four general chemical classes: strongly acidic, weakly acidic, basic, and neutral compounds. The majority of the mass in each case was in the neutral fraction (63 to 92%). The other classes expressed the following ranges: basic (1.67 to 25%), weakly acidic (3.5 to 12%), and strongly acidic (2.9 to 6.3%). These various extracts and fractions were examined for mutagenic activity by several test systems including the *Salmonella*/mammalian microsome reversion assay.

There is a wide range of response of the *Salmonella* strains to a given quantity of a mutagenic compound. As demonstrated by Johnston and Hopke,[63] the response per unit weight varies over six orders of magnitude so that a small response may be the result of a large quantity of a weak mutagen or a small quantity of a potent agent. Also, a weak response

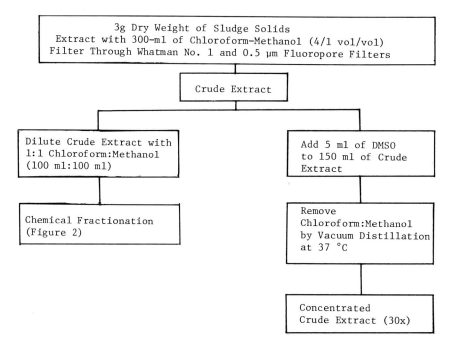

FIGURE 1.   Outline of the modified extraction protocol.

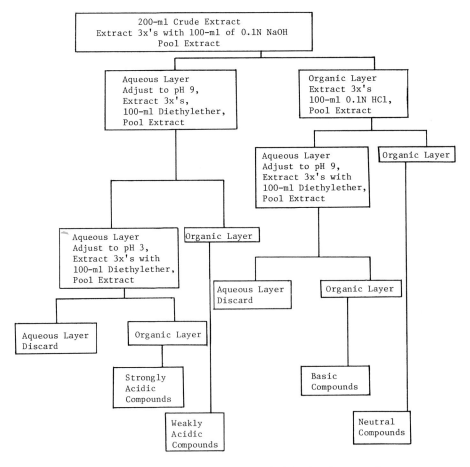

FIGURE 2.   Schematic outline of the chemical fractionation protocol.

is not an indication that an agent is harmless. There are potent carcinogens such as the nitrosamines that show low activity in the *Salmonella* strains. This difference in sensitivity emphasizes the need for a multiorganism testing approach as recommended by the U.S. Environmental Protection Agency.[64]

The *Salmonella*/mammalian microsome reversion assay employing strains TA98 and TA100 used the top agar incorporation procedure described by Ames et al.[65] and incorporated the recommendations of de Serres and Shelby.[66] TA98 and TA100 were chosen because they are the most sensitive and respond to the widest range of chemical classes. Mammalian activation of the test agents was included by using a standard S9 mix. The hepatic S9 fraction was prepared as described by Ames et al.[65] from male Sprague-Dawley rats induced with either Aroclor 1254 or phenobarbital. The purpose of adding S9 to the assay was to simulate mammalian metabolism of test agents and to detect promutagens, compounds that become mutagenically active as a result of metabolism.

In the *Salmonella* assay, the response to a mutagenic compound would result in a curve where the number of his[+] revertants increased with increasing concentration to the point where, on the average, one lethal mutation per cell has occurred. From that point there will be a decline in response due to the accumulation of deleterious mutations leading to the death of the test organism. In complex mixtures such as these extracts, there can also be direct toxicity to the organism superimposed on the mutagenic response curve.

The mutagenic activities of the aqueous supernatant liquids assayed with *Salmonella* are presented in Table 7. Fractions A1 and A2b did not show the presence of any direct-acting mutagens. Fraction A2a produced equivocal responses in TA98 with Aroclor/S9 activation and in TA100 without activation. Therefore, no mutagenic activities were associated with the aqueous supernatant liquid.

The results of the extracts of the sludge pellet are also presented in Table 7. Direct acting mutagens were not detected in extracts E1 or E2. With the addition of the Aroclor/S9 mix, these fractions exhibited a mutagenic response. The equivalent of 0.6 $\mu\ell$ of E1 produced an approximate doubling in the number of revertant colonies per plate. The elevated but flat response of the assay to extract E2 precluded estimation of a doubling dose. This dose-response behavior illustrates the difficulties of analyzing complex mixtures.

The successive extraction of mutagenic compound(s) by acetone from the sludge pellet is presented in Table 8. The mutagenic activity recovered in fractions F1 and F2 was approximately the same for both TA98 and TA100. The mutagenic activity present in F3 was less than in fractions F1 and F2. When assayed with TA100, fractions F1 and F2 were more toxic per volume of extract than fraction F3 since there were lower numbers of revertant colonies observed for the higher doses assayed. The amount of the pellet dissolved by the acetone increased in each successive extraction. Therefore, the amount of mutagenic activity per milligram of acetone-soluble material decreased with each extraction. It is apparent that fraction F1 had the highest mutagenicity to mass ratio of the three fractions.

Subsequently, the crude chloroform:methanol extracts from all five samples, Champaign, Chicago, Hinsdale, Kankakee, and Sauget, were examined for mutation induction. The data are presented in Table 9. The Sauget crude extract was very mutagenic. Both in the absence or presence of Aroclor/S9, linear dose-dependent responses were induced by the Sauget crude extract. A doubling over the control in the number of revertants per plate was induced by 139 μg of Sauget crude extract residue. The slopes of the responses indicated that the Sauget crude extract residue induced 260 revertants per milligram without S9 and 780 revertants per milligram with Aroclor/S9. The presence of Aroclor/S9 enhanced the yield of revertants per milligram of residue by a factor of three.

The Champaign, Chicago, Hinsdale, and Kankakee crude extracts did not induce a doubling over the control or a dose-dependent increase in the number of revertants per plate. Therefore, these crude extracts were not directly mutagenic. These extracts demonstrated a negative response with either type of S9.

Table 7
MUTAGENICITY OF POOLED EXTRACTS OF CHICAGO SEWAGE SLUDGE USING AMES STRAINS TA98 AND TA100

						TA98		TA100	
Sample	Vol/plate (μℓ)	Dilution factor	Equivalent vol/plate (μℓ)	Concentration factor (V/V)	Equivalent vol of neat sludge/ plate (μℓ)	−S9	+S9	−S9	+S9
DMSO	100						57 ± 23[a]		
E1	10	0.02	0.2	325	65		89 ± 17		
	20	0.02	0.4		130		100 ± 15		
	30	0.02	0.6		195		131 ± 17		
	40	0.02	0.8		260		133 ± 19		
	50	0.02	1.0		325		136 ± 21		
E2	10	0.1	1.0	260	260		89 ± 24		
	20	0.1	2.0		520		103 ± 25		
	30	0.1	3.0		780		109 ± 21		
	50	0.1	5.0		1,300		117 ± 29		
	100	0.1	10.0		2,600		100 ± 12		
Water	2,000					60 ± 5[b]	80 ± 6	155 ± 3	184 ± 8
A1	100		100	1.25	125	69 ± 7	86 ± 10	165 ± 10	192 ± 8
	300	1.0	300		375	63 ± 1	90 ± 2	167 ± 18	192 ± 4
	2,000	1.0	2,000		2,500	67 ± 20	79 ± 6	161 ± 4	174 ± 2
DMSO	100					31 ± 1	70 ± 21	115 ± 7	130 ± 7
A2a	50	0.1	5	125	625	37 ± 1	72 ± 11	131 ± 16	103 ± 10
	100	0.1	10		1,250	29 ± 1	59 ± 13	143 ± 17	114 ± 4
	20	1.0	20		2,500	35 ± 8	55 ± 9	146 ± —	140 ± 17
	50	1.0	50		6,250	39 ± 0	60 ± 23	140 ± 40	146 ± 2
	100	1.0	100		12,500	37 ± —	95 ± 45	173 ± 8	154 ± 6
A2b	50	0.1	5	125	625	29 ± 2	44 ± 15	115 ± 9	108 ± 13
	100	0.1	10		1,250	35 ± 1	50 ± 3	139 ± 24	125 ± 25
	20	1.0	20		2,500	42 ± 5	55 ± 13	127 ± 18	135 ± 7
	50	1.0	50		6,250	36 ± 6	nd	156 ± 16	153 ± 17
	100	1.0	100		12,500	41 ± 1	nd	146 ± 12	148 ± 17

Note: nd indicates that a value was not determined.

[a] Data are derived from triplicate platings.
[b] Data are derived from duplicate platings.

Table 8
MUTAGENICITY OF THE THREE SEQUENTIAL ACETONE EXTRACTIONS OF CHICAGO SEWAGE SLUDGE IN AMES STRAINS TA98 AND TA100 FOLLOWING AROCLOR/S9 ACTIVATION

Sample	Vol/plate (μℓ)	Dilution factor	Equivalent vol/plate (μℓ)	Concentration (mg/mℓ)	Mass/plate (mg)	TA98 revertants/plate	TA100 revertants/plate
Control	100			0.0	0.0	52 ± 6	130 ± 7
F1	50	1	50	2.1	0.1	76 ± 6	162 ± 12
	100	1	100	2.1	0.2	97 ± 9	218 ± 11
	20	10	200	2.1	0.4	160 ± 11	254 ± 1
	50	10	500	2.1	1.0	225 ± 28	280 ± 3
	100	10	1000	2.1	2.1	nd	68 ± 23
F2	50	1	50	7.3	0.4	83 ± 1	164 ± 4
	100	1	100	7.3	0.7	110 ± 20	235 ± 24
	20	10	200	7.3	1.5	144 ± 30	284 ± 1
	50	10	500	7.3	3.7	164 ± 7	297 ± 20
	100	10	1000	7.3	7.3	nd	172 ± 13
F3	50	1	50	23.9	1.2	57 ± 6	166 ± 18
	100	1	100	23.9	2.4	78 ± 9	171 ± 13
	20	10	200	23.9	4.8	93 ± 11	208 ± 14
	50	10	500	23.9	12.0	124 ± 13	253 ± 11
	100	10	1000	23.9	23.9	nd	287 ± 35

Note: nd indicates that a value was not determined.

Table 9

MUTAGENICITY OF CRUDE CHLOROFORM:METHANOL EXTRACTS IN TA98 IN THE ABSENCE AND PRESENCE OF S9

Sample	Vol (μℓ)	Conc. factor	Mass equiv. vol (μℓ)	Conc. (mg/mℓ)	Conc./plate (μg)	Revertants/plate −S9	+S9[a]	+S9[b]
CHMP	100	—	100	0	0.0	25	60	32
	100	0.1	10	650	6.5	31	50	40
		1.0	100		65.0	25	50	48
		10.0	1000		650.0	36	29	31
		30.0	3000		1900.0	K[c]	K	34
CHI	100	—	100	0	0.0	21	58	40
	100	0.1	10	770	7.7	22	55	32
		1.0	100		77.0	18	58	39
		10.0	1000		770.0	26	35	65
		30.0	3000		2300.0	K	18	42
HNSD	100	—	100	0	0.0	27	71	40
	100	0.1	10	470	4.7	25	71	47
		1.0	100		47.0	36	68	55
		10.0	1000		470.0	45	74	57
		30.0	3000		1400.0	41	64	63
KANK	100	—	100	0	0.0	23	61	
	100	0.1	10	1250	12.5	25	56	
		1.0	100		125.0	29	42	
		10.0	1000		1250.0	27	38	
		30.0	3000		3750.0	K	K	
SAUG	100	—	100	0	0.0	28	66	
	100	0.1	10	1390	13.9	30	79	
		1.0	100		139.0	61	214	
		10.0	1000		1390.0	377	741	
		30.0	3000		4170.0	1137	3363	

[a] Aroclor/S9.
[b] Phenobarbital/S9.
[c] K: absence or partial absence of bacterial lawn as an indicator of toxicity.

The results of the mutation assays of each subfraction are presented in Table 10. The concentration of each fraction was low. Thus, fractions were tested at the lower limits of resolution. The slopes of the dose-dependent response were determined for only those fractions that demonstrated: (1) a doubling over the control in the number of revertants per plate and (2) a dose-dependent response with a minimum of two doses that equaled or exceeded a doubling over the control.

The neutral fractions of the Champaign, Chicago, and Hinsdale extracts did not demonstrate a mutagenic response in TA98 with or without S9 mix. Those fractions that did induce a weak or clear mutagenic response were the basic, strongly acidic, and weakly acidic fractions. S9 did not enhance the mutagenic activity of these extracts.

All the Sauget fractions induced a mutagenic response in TA98 (Table 10). The basic fraction was the most mutagenic (1600 revertants per milligram residue) and the weakly acidic was the least mutagenic (27.6 revertants per milligram residue). Both the neutral and strongly acidic fractions were very mutagenic, 129 and 380 revertants per milligram residue, respectively.

The Sauget sample has substantially different properties than any of the other samples. With Aroclor/S9, the basic fraction was the most mutagenic. However, the Aroclor/S9 eliminated the mutagenic response exhibited by the weakly acidic fraction. Thus, both the

Table 10
MUTAGENICITY OF MUNICIPAL SEWAGE SLUDGE SUBFRACTIONS IN TA98 WITH AND WITHOUT S9

Sample	Vol (μℓ)	Conc. factor	Mass equiv. vol (μℓ)	Conc. (mg/mℓ)	Conc./plate (μg)	Revertants/plate		
						− S9	+ S9[a]	+ S9[b]
CHMP neutr.	100	0	0	0	0	24	53	32
	50	3.0	50	199	29.9	29	34	36
	100	3.0	300		59.7	26	52	32
	50	30.0	1500		299.0	27	48	39
	100	30.0	3000		597.0	19	39	41
Bases	100	0	0	0	0	24	53	32
	50	3.0	150	79.5	11.9	25	47	54
	100	3.0	300		23.9	34	54	59
	50	30.0	1500		119.0	64	51	50
	100	30.0	3000		239.0	97	99	69
Weak acids	100	0	0	0	0	24	53	32
	50	3.0	150	38.2	5.7	27	58	40
	100	3.0	300		11.5	40	54	43
	50	30.0	1500		57.3	50	88	67
	100	30.0	3000		115.0	60	88	71
Strong acids	100	0	0	0	0	24	53	32
	50	3.0	150			32	44	40
	100	3.0	300			34	58	41
	50	30.0	1500			71	109	72
	100	30.0	3000			116	119	100
CHI neutr.	100	0	0	0	0	16	49	40
	50	3.0	150	294	44.0	19	57	39
	100	3.0	300		88.0	17	64	45
	50	30.0	1500		441.0	26	60	37
	100	30.0	3000		882.0	14	53	36
Bases	100	0	0	0	0	16	49	40
	50	3.0	150	53.2	8.0	23	63	22
	100	3.0	300		16.0	26	59	34
	50	30.0	1500		80.0	66	70	40
	100	30.0	3000		160.0	58	76	40
Weak acids	100	0	0	0	0	16	49	40
	50	3.0	150	26.4	3.0	22	65	36
	100	3.0	300		6.1	15	87	41
	50	30.0	1500		30.0	38	66	41
	100	30.0	3000		61.0	38	66	41
Strong acids	100	0	0	0	0	16	49	40
	50	3.0	150	25.0	3.8	20	64	31
	100	3.0	300		7.6	25	67	37
	50	30.0	1500		38.0	49	94	36
	100	30.0	3000		76.0	53	99	63
HNSD neutr.	100	0	0	0	0	32	85	40
	50	3.0	150			30	93	47
	100	3.0	300			31	100	36
	50	30.0	1500				116	43
	100	30.0	3000			39	106	60
Bases	100	0	0	0	0	32	85	40
	50	3.0	150	17.9	2.7	31	95	32
	100	3.0	300		5.4	31	93	35
	50	30.0	1500		27.0	58	93	43
	100	30.0	3000		52.0	58	103	65
Weak acids	100	0	0	0	0	32	85	40
	50	3.0	150	38.2	4.7	24	84	39

Table 10 (continued)
MUTAGENICITY OF MUNICIPAL SEWAGE SLUDGE SUBFRACTIONS IN TA98 WITH AND WITHOUT S9

Sample	Vol (μℓ)	Conc. factor	Mass equiv. vol (μℓ)	Conc. (mg/mℓ)	Conc./plate (μg)	Revertants/plate		
						−S9	+S9[a]	+S9[b]
	100	3.0	300		9.4	36	90	39
	50	30.0	1500		47.0	82	305	66
	100	30.0	3000		94.0	79	113	67
Strong acids	100	0	0	0	0	32	85	40
	50	3.0	150	31.6	4.8	32	83	41
	100	3.0	300		9.6	32	72	49
	50	30.0	1500		48.0	69	97	67
	100	30.0	3000		96.0	94	112	—
SAUG neutr.	100	0	0	0	0	31	66	
	50	3.0	150	525	7.8	31	66	
	100	30.0	100		158.0	84	214	
	50	30.0	1500		788.0	145	293	
	100	30.0	3000		1580.0	253	488	
Bases	100	0	0	0	0	31	66	
	50	3.0	150	19.7	2.9	37	76	
	100	3.0	300		5.8	49	68	
	50	30.0	1500		29.0	78	80	
	100	30.0	3000		58.0	127	130	
Weak acids	100	0	0	0	0	31	66	
	50	3.0	150	51.8	7.8	31	66	
	100	3.0	300		15.5	39	61	
	50	30.0	1500		780.0	52	50	
	100	30.0	3000		1550.0	77	76	
Strong acids	100	0	0	0	0	31	66	
	50	3.0	150	33.6	5.0	49	55	
	100	3.0	300		30.0	30.0	59	
	50	30.0	1500		50.0	57	78	
	100	30.0	3000		301.0	73	101	

[a] Aroclor/S9.
[b] Phenobarbital/S9.

basic and weakly acidic fractions exhibited a decreased yield of revertants per milligram residue that demonstrated a net metabolic deactivation of mutagens into nonmutagens. The neutral and strongly acidic fractions were very mutagenic and exhibited an enhanced yield of revertants with Aroclor/S9. With Aroclor/S9, the neutral fraction induced 248 revertants per milligram residue, whereas this fraction alone induced 129 revertants per milligram residue. The mutagenic activity of the neutral fraction was enhanced 1.9-fold (248 revertants per milligram residue per 129 revertants per milligram residue) by Aroclor/S9. Similarly, the strongly acidic fraction exhibited an enhanced mutagenic activity with Aroclor/S9. With Aroclor/S9, the strongly acidic fraction induced 480 revertants per milligram residue whereas without Aroclor/S9, this fraction induced 320 revertants per milligram residue representing a 1.1-fold enhancement. The mutation frequency per milligram of residue induced by the crude extract was enhanced threefold by Aroclor/S9, and the sum of the Aroclor/S9 enhanced mutagenicity for the neutral and the strongly acidic fractions was threefold. Therefore, the net effect of the metabolism of promutagens to ultimate mutagens by Aroclor/S9 can be accounted for by the net effects of the neutral and strongly acidic fractions.

If the effects of these Sauget fractions were independent, then the sum of the normalized reverse-mutation frequencies should approximately equal the reverse-mutation frequency

Table 11
MUTAGENICITY OF SAUGET FRACTIONS IN
TA98 WITH AND WITHOUT S9

Fraction	Normalized no. of revertants/mg of residue		Crude extract (%)	Revertants/mg of residue	
	− S9	+ S9		− S9	+ S9
Neutral	129	248	83.4	108	207
Basic	1,600	10,000	3.1	50	31
Weakly acidic	27.6	—	8.2	2	—
Strongly acidic	380	420	5.3	20	22
Total				180	260
Crude	260	780	100	260	780

induced by the crude extract. Table 11 presents the mutagenic activity and a normalized value for the mutation frequencies for each fraction with and without Aroclor/S9. The sum of the normalized direct acting mutagenicity of these fractions equaled 180 revertants per milligram of residue, whereas the crude extract induced 260 revertants per milligram of residue. These data suggest that these fractions act independently of each other. In the presence of Aroclor/S9, the crude extract induced threefold more revertants per milligram of residue than the sum of the normalized mutation frequencies of the individual extracts. This indicates that these fractions are more mutagenic in the crude extract than as separate entities, suggesting the presence of a synergistic effect(s).

III. CONCLUSIONS

Although a component of the mutagens present in municipal sewage sludge must be naturally occurring compounds, there exist in such complex mixtures a wide variety of synthetic chemicals of anthropogenic origin. The differences of the various sewage sludges cannot merely reflect the presence of naturally occurring agents. The general mutagenic potency of a sludge appears to be related to the industrial activity of the area that contributes to the sewage treatment facility. Ellis and co-workers[67] have detected a wide range of toxic organic components in effluents from publicly owned treatment facilities in Illinois. Of the tentative identification of 243 compounds, 20 compounds are listed by the U.S. Environmental Protection Agency as priority pollutants. The publicly owned treatment facilities that were involved in the study were located in Addison, Bartlett, Bensenville, Danville, Decatur, Roselle, and Sauget, Illinois. Among the agents contained in one or more of the effluents were aromatic hydrocarbons, phenols, plasticizers, halogenated compounds, anilines, indoles, and s-triazine herbicides.

The presence of naturally occurring mutagens in sewage sludge may pose some environmental hazard. However, there may exist a background level of naturally occurring mutagens in all sewage sludges. It seems prudent to identify those waste treatment plants that discharge effluents significantly more mutagenic than what would be expected from naturally occurring agents. It is reasonable to regulate the discharge of synthetic chemical mutagens into a publicly owned treatment facility prior to their release into the environment.

REFERENCES

1. **Hinesly, T. D. and Sosewitz, B.,** Digested sludge disposal on crop land, *J. Water Pollut. Control Fed.,* 41, 882, 1969.
2. **Hinesly, T. D., Braids, O. C., Dick, R. I., Jones, R. L., and Molina, J. A. E.,** Agricultural Benefits and Environmental Changes Resulting from the Use of Digested Sludge on Field Crops, Report D01-UI-00080, U.S. Environmental Protection Agency, Cincinnati, 1974.
3. **Hinesly, T. D., Jones, R. L., and Ziegler E. L.,** Effect on corn by applications of heated anaerobically digested sludge, *Compost. Sci.,* 13, 26, 1972.
4. **Varanka, M. W., Zablocki, Z. M., and Hinesly, T. D.,** Effect of digested sewage sludge on biological activity in soil, *J. Water Pollut. Control Fed.,* 48, 1728, 1976.
5. **Hinesly, T. D., Jones, R. D., Ziegler, E. L., and Tayler, J. J.,** Effect of annual and accumulated applications of sewage sludge on assimilation of zinc and cadmium by corn (*Zea mays* L.), *Environ. Sci. Technol.,* 11, 182, 1977.
6. **Hinesly, T. D., Alexander, D. E., Ziegler, E. L., and Barrett, G. L.,** Zinc and Cd accumulation by corn inbreds grown on sludge amended soil, *Agron. J.,* 70, 425, 1978.
7. **Freese, E.,** Genetic effects of mutagens and of agents present in the human environment, in *Molecular and Environmental Aspects of Mutagenesis,* Prakash, L., Ed., Charles C Thomas, Springfield, Ill., 1974, 5.
8. **de Serres, F. J.,** Long-range planning for effective *in vitro* tests for carcinogenesis, in *Screening Tests in Chemical Carcinogenesis,* IARC Sci. Publ. No. 12, Montesano, R., Bartsch, H., and Tomatis, H., Eds., International Agency for Research on Cancer, Lyon, France, 1976, 29.
9. **Ames, B. N.,** Identifying environmental chemicals causing mutations and cancer, *Science,* 204, 587, 1979.
10. **Crow, J. F.,** Impact of various types of genetic damage and risk assessment, in *Environmental Health Perspectives,* Experimental Issue No. 6, de Serres, F. J. and Sheridan, W., Eds., U.S. National Institutes of Health, Bethesda, Md., 1973, 1.
11. **Hemminki, K., Saloniemi, I., Luoma, K., Salonen, T., Partanen, T., Vainio, H., and Hemminki, E.,** Transplacental carcinogens and mutagens: childhood cancer, malformations and abortions as risk indicators, *J. Toxicol. Environ. Health,* 6, 1115, 1980.
12. **Benditt, E. P.,** The origin of atherosclerosis, *Sci. Am.,* 235, 74, 1977.
13. **Epstein, C. J. and Globus, M. S.,** Prenatal diagnosis of genetic diseases, *Am. Sci.,* 65, 703, 1977.
14. **Heidelberger, C.,** Chemical carcinogenesis, *Annu. Rev. Biochem.,* 44, 79, 1975.
15. **Bouck, N. and di Mayorca, G.,** Somatic mutation as the basis for malignant transformation of BHK cells by chemical carcinogens, *Nature (London),* 264, 722, 1976.
16. **Sorsa, M.,** Somatic mutation theory, *J. Toxicol. Environ. Health,* 6, 57, 1980.
17. **Epstein, S. S.,** Environmental determinants of human cancer, *Cancer Res.,* 34, 2425, 1974.
18. **Ong, T. and de Serres, F. J.,** Mutagenicity of chemical carcinogens in *Neurospora crassa, Cancer Res.,* 32, 1890, 1972.
19. **de Serres, F. J.,** The correlation between carcinogenic and mutagenic activity in short-term tests for mutation-induction and DNA repair, *Mutat. Res.,* 31, 203, 1975.
20. **McCann, J., Choi, E., Yamasaki, E., and Ames, B. N.,** Detection of carcinogens as mutagens in the *Salmonella*/microsome test: assay of 300 chemicals, *Proc. Natl. Acad. Sci. U.S.A.,* 72, 5135, 1975.
21. **McCann, J. and Ames, B. N.,** Detection of carcinogens as mutagens in the *Salmonella*/microsome test: assay of 300 chemicals. Discussion, *Proc. Natl. Acad. Sci. U.S.A.,* 73, 950, 1976.
22. **Sugimura, T., Sato, S., Nago, M., Yahaggi, T., Matsushima, T., Senio, Y., Takenchi, M., and Kawaehi, T.,** Overlapping of carcinogens and mutagens, in *Fundamentals in Cancer Prevention,* Magee, P. N., Ed., University Park Press, Baltimore, 1976, 191.
23. **Purchase, I. F. H., Longstaff, E., Ashby, J., Styles, J. A., Anderson, D., Lefevre, P. A., and Westwood, F. R.,** Evaluation of six short-term tests for potential carcinogenicity and recommendations for their use, *Nature (London),* 264, 624, 1976.
24. **Harrington, W. M., Jr.,** Hazardous solid waste from domestic wastewater treatment plants, *Environ. Health Perspect.,* 27, 231, 1978.
25. **Neuffer, M. G., Jones, L., and Zuber, M. S.,** *The Mutants of Maize,* Crop Science Society of America, Madison, Wis., 1968, 5.
26. **Lehninger, A. L.,** *Biochemistry,* Worth Publishing, New York, 1970, 229.
27. **Plewa, M. J.,** Activation of chemicals into mutagens by green plants: a preliminary discussion, *Environ. Health Perspect.,* 27, 45, 1978.
28. **Gentile, J. M., Gentile, G. J., Bultman, J., Sechriest, R., Wagner, E. D., and Plewa, M. J.,** An evaluation of the genotoxic properties of insecticides following plant and animal activation, *Mutat. Res.,* 101, 19, 1982.
29. **Plewa, M. J. and Wagner, E. D.,** Germinal cell mutagenesis in specially designed maize genotypes, *Environ. Health Perspect.,* 37, 61, 1981.

30. **Bianchi, A.,** Some aspects of mutagenesis in maize, *Mutat. Process Proc. Symp.,* 30, 1965.
31. **Hodgdon, A. L., Marcus, A. H., Arenaz, P., Rosichan, J. L., Bogyo, T. P., and Nilan, R. A.,** Ontogeny of the barley plant as related to mutation expression and detection of pollen mutations, *Environ. Health Perspect.,* 37, 5, 1981.
32. **Constantin, M. J. and Nilan, R. A.,** The chlorophyll-deficient mutant assay in barley *(Hordeum vulgare):* a report of the U.S. Environmental Protection Agency Gene-Tox Program, *Mutat. Res.,* 99, 1, 1982.
33. **Plewa, M. J. and Dowd, P. A.,** Induction of forward mutation in somatic cells of maize after acute or chronic exposure to ethylmethanesulfonate, *Maize Genet. Coop. Newslett.,* 56, 157, 1982.
34. **Plewa, M. J.,** Specific locus mutation assays in *Zea mays:* a report of the U.S. Environmental Protection Agency Gene-Tox Program, *Mutat. Res.,* 99, 317, 1982.
35. **Freeling, M.,** Maize *Adh1* as a monitor of environmental mutagens, *Environ. Health Perspect.,* 27, 91, 1978.
36. **Freeling, M.,** Toward monitoring specific DNA lesions in the gene by using pollen systems, *Environ. Health Perspect.,* 37, 13, 1981.
37. **Schwartz, D.,** *Adh* locus in maize for detection of mutagens in the environment, *Environ. Health Perspect.,* 37, 75, 1981.
38. **Vig, B. K.,** Somatic mosaicism in plants with special reference to somatic crossing over, *Environ. Health Perspect.,* 27, 27, 1978.
39. **Vig, B. K.,** Soybean *(Glycine max* [L.] Merrill) as a short-term assay for study of environmental mutagens: a report of the U.S. Environmental Protection Agency Gene-Tox Program, *Mutat. Res.,* 99, 339, 1982.
40. **Schairer, L. A., Van't Hof, J., Hayes, C. G., Burton, R. M., and de Serres, F. J.,** Exploratory monitoring of air pollutants for mutagenicity activity with the *Tradescantia* stamen hair system, *Environ. Health Perspect.,* 27, 51, 1978.
41. **Ma, T. H.,** Tradescantia micronucleus bioassay and pollen tube chromatid aberration test for *in situ* monitoring and mutagen screening, *Environ. Health Perspect.,* 37, 85, 1981.
42. **Ma, T. H.,** *Tradescantia* cytogenetic tests (root tip mitosis, pollen mitosis, pollen mother cell meiosis): a report of the U.S. Environmental Protection Agency Gene-Tox Program, *Mutat. Res.,* 99, 293, 1982.
43. **Hopke, P. K., Plewa, M. J., Johnston, J. B., Weaver, D., Wood, S. G., Larson, R. A., and Hinesly, T.,** Multitechnique screening of Chicago municipal sewage sludge for mutagenic activity, *Environ. Sci. Technol.,* 16, 140, 1982.
44. **Hoagland, D. R. and Arnon, D. I.,** California Agriculture Experimental Station Circular No. 347, 1950.
45. **Epler, J. L.,** The use of short-term tests in the isolation and identification of chemical mutagens in complex mixtures, in *Chemical Mutagens: Principles and Methods for Their Detection,* Vol. 6, de Serres, F. J. and Hollaender, A., Eds., Plenum Press, New York, 1980, 239.
46. **Kier, L. D., Yamasaki, E., and Ames, B. N.,** Detection of mutagenic activity in cigarette smoke condensates, *Proc. Natl. Acad. Sci. U.S.A.,* 71, 4159, 1974.
47. **Hutton, J. J. and Hackney, C.,** Metabolism of cigarette smoke condensates by human and rat homogenates to form mutagens detectable by *Salmonella typhimurium* TA1538, *Cancer Res.,* 35, 2461, 1975.
48. **Yamasaki, E. and Ames, B. N.,** Concentration of mutagens from urine by absorption with the nonpolar resin XAD-2: cigarette smokers have mutagenic urine, *Proc. Natl. Acad. Sci. U.S.A.,* 74, 3555, 1977.
49. **Hardigree, A. A. and Epler, J. L.,** Mutagenicity of plant flavonols in microbial systems, *Mutat. Res.,* 53, 89, 1978.
50. **Plewa, M. J. and Gentile, J. M.,** The activation of chemicals into mutagens by green plants, in *Chemical Mutagens: Principles and Methods for Their Detection,* Vol. 7, de Serres, F. J. and Hollaender, A., Eds., Plenum Press, New York, 1982, 401.
51. **Sugimura, T.,** A view of a cancer researcher on environmental mutagens, in *Environmental Mutagens and Carcinogens,* Sugimura, T., Kondo, S., and Takebe, H., Eds., Alan R. Liss, New York, 1982, 7.
52. **Stich, H. F., Wu, C., and Powrie, W.,** Enhancement and suppression of genotoxicity of foods by naturally occurring components in these products, in *Environmental Mutagens and Carcinogens,* Sugimura, T., Kondo, S., and Takebe, H., Eds., Alan R. Liss, New York, 1982, 347.
53. **Ames, B. N., Kammen, H. O., and Yamasaki, E.,** Hair dyes are mutagenic: identification of a variety of mutagenic ingredients, *Proc. Natl. Acad. Sci. U.S.A.,* 72, 2432, 1975.
54. **Neubert, D.,** Nature and levels of chemical environmental mutagens, industrial exposure and population at risk, in *Progress in Genetic Toxicology,* Scott, D., Bridges, B. A., and Sobels, F. H., Eds., Elsevier/North Holland, New York, 1977, 95.
55. **Chrisp, C. E., Fisher, G. L., and Lammert, J. E.,** Mutagenicity of filtrates from respirable coal fly ash, *Science,* 199, 73, 1978.
56. **Pitts, J. N., Jr., Grosjeru, D., Mischke, T. M., Simmons, V. F., and Poole, D.,** Mutagenic activity of airborne particulate organic pollutants, *Toxicol. Lett.,* 1, 65, 1977.
57. **Commoner, B., Madyastha, P., Bronsdon, A., and Vithayathil, A. J.,** Environmental mutagens in urban air particles, *J. Toxicol. Environ. Health,* 4, 59, 1978.

58. **Dehnen, W., Ritz, N., and Tomingas, R.,** The mutagenicity of airborne particulate pollutants, *Cancer Lett.,* 4, 5, 1977.

59. **Teranishi, K., Hamada, K., and Watanabe, H.,** Mutagenicity in *Salmonella typhimurium* mutants of the benzene-soluble organic matter derived from airborne particulate matter and its five fractions, *Mutat. Res.,* 56, 273, 1978.

60. **Durston, W. E. and Ames, B. N.,** A simple method for the detection of mutagens in urine: studies with the carcinogen 2-acetylaminofluorene, *Proc. Natl. Acad. Sci. U.S.A.,* 71, 737, 1974.

61. **San, R. H. C., Stich, H. F., Acton, A. B., and Maus, L.,** Human sewage: a source of environmental mutagens? *Environ. Mutagenesis,* 3, 350, 1981.

62. **Junk, G. A., Richards, J. J., Greiner, M. D., Wittiak, D., Arguello, M. D., Vick, R., Svec, H. J., Fritz, J. S., and Calder, G. V.,** Use of macroreticular resins in the analysis of water for trace organic contaminants, *J. Chromatogr.,* 99, 745, 1974.

63. **Johnston, J. B. and Hopke, P. K.,** Estimation of the weight-dependent probability of detecting a mutagen with the Ames assay, *Environ. Mutagenesis,* 2, 419, 1980.

64. U.S. Environmental Protection Agency, Environmental Assessment, Short-Term Tests for Carcinogens, Mutagens and Other Genotoxic Agents, EPA-625/9-79-003, Environmental Research Information Center, USEPA, Cincinnati, 1979.

65. **Ames, B. N., McCann, J., and Yamasaki, E.,** Methods for detecting carcinogens and mutagens with the *Salmonella* mammalian-microsome mutagenicity test, *Mutat. Res.,* 31, 347, 1975.

66. **de Serres, F. J. and Shelby, M. D.,** The *Salmonella* mutagenicity assay: recommendations, *Science,* 203, 563, 1979.

67. **Ellis, D. D., Jones, C. M., Larson, R. A., and Schaeffer, D. J.,** Organic constituents of mutagenic secondary effluents from wastewater treatment plants, *Arch. Environ. Contaminants Toxicol.,* 11, 373, 1982.

Chapter 17

MUTAGENIC ACTIVITY IN AGRICULTURAL SOILS

Waltraud Göggelmann and Peter Spitzauer

TABLE OF CONTENTS

I. INTRODUCTION

In the past few years various studies have reported that investigations on complex environmental mixtures lead to the detection of mutagenic activity in water,[1,2] airborne particles,[3] and food.[4] In several cases mutagenic activity has contributed to the presence of polycyclic aromatic hydrocarbons (PAH), especially in airborne particles,[5] which can sediment to soil. In 1961 Blumer[6] reported that the carcinogen benzo[a]pyrene was found in soils and further investigations were carried out to determine the content of PAH in soils from various parts of the world.[7-9] However, studies on mutagenic activity in soils have not been reported so far. Therefore, we studied the mutagenic activity in agricultural soils and tried to assess responsible sources for the mutagenic activity.

II. MATERIALS AND METHODS

The soil samples were derived from a rural, low-density traffic area of about 30 km² in southern Germany. Hops and asparagus were cultivated within the last years on the same fields, whereas cereal growing changed from year to year. All soil samples were collected in the spring, taken at a depth of 0 to 10 cm at several points of a few agricultural fields, and thoroughly mixed. Information on the types and amounts of fertilizers and pesticides frequently used within the last years have been provided by the farmers. The content of humus was determined by the method of Springer and Klee.[10]

Mutagenicity of the soil samples was analyzed by the method of Ames et al.[11] The tests were performed with and without addition of Clophen A50-activated liver S9 from Wistar rats with the *Salmonella typhimurium* strains TA98 and TA100. A method extracting the soil samples for mutagenicity tests was developed. Moist soil samples were ($\sim$24 hr) soxhlet-extracted with hexane/acetone overnight. The extracts were carefully evaporated to small volumes under nitrogen and after 12 hr centrifuged for 20 min at 2000 xg. The resulting supernatants were mixed with supernatants, received after suspension of the pellets in isopropanol/DMSO and subsequent centrifugation, and then concentrated. DMSO was added until all precipitated material had been solubilized. One hundred grams (100 g) soil corresponded to approximately 1 mℓ extract, of which aliquots were used for mutagenicity testing.

High performance liquid chromatography (HPLC)[12] was used in a modified version to screen for the PAH. To separate other interfering organic matter from the PAH fraction, moist soil samples were extracted twice with hexane/acetone. Extracts were filtered through an Na_2SO_4/quartz sand column, evaporated, and chromatographed on a silica gel HPLC column. The main fraction was mixed with isopropanol, evaporated, and characterized at a fluorescence detector. Peaks observed in the sample chromatographic profiles were compared with the retention times of known standards. All peak areas within the retention range of anthracene to 1,2,4,5-dibenzpyrene were estimated and the total PAH content was calculated with the response factor of fluoranthene.

III. RESULTS AND DISCUSSION

The results of mutagenicity testing obtained with TA98 and TA100 and different amounts of soil extracts from several asparagus cultures and meadows are shown in Figure 1. Only small differences in the number of induced revertants were observed. Results obtained with soil samples of different cultures in the presence and absence of S9 mix are shown in Figure 2. Survival was 80 to 100% for all soil samples (data not shown). In TA98, significant mutagenicity was induced by soil extracts of hops and asparagus cultures which showed 9-fold higher numbers of induced than spontaneous revertants. When testing soil extracts of rye, oat, pasture, and meadow, lower yields of induced revertants were obtained. With S9 mix, mutagenicity in TA98 was in an equal order as without S9 mix. TA100 showed less

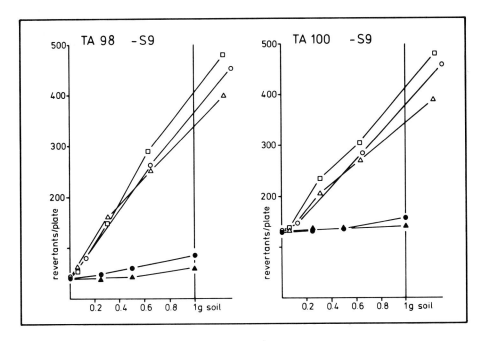

FIGURE 1. Dose-response curves of agricultural soil extracts. Different amounts of soil extracts were assayed with *Salmonella* strains TA98 and TA100 without S9 mix. Each point gives the mean value of three plates of one representative experiment out of three. Soil extracts of different asparagus cultures ○, △,□ and meadows ●,▲.

mutagenicity than TA98. With soil extracts of hops and asparagus cultures, the number of induced revertants per gram of soil was only 3 times higher than the control values if tested without S9 mix. A remarkable increase in mutagenicity was observed when testing soil extracts of hops, asparagus, and meadow in the presence of S9 mix. However, it can be stated that all tested soils showed mutagenic activity and that in particular, an increased mutagenicity was observed in soils of special cultures (hops, asparagus).

The major source of the mutagenic activity in the tested soil samples may be that man has introduced mutagens and carcinogens into the environment. However, the existence of natural mutagens is known for fungi containing aflatoxins[13] or for higher plants containing pyrrolizidine alkaloids,[13] flavonoids,[14] and benzoxazinones.[15] Hops and asparagus exhibiting the highest mutagenicity in soil extracts belong to the families of Cannabaceae and Liliaceae which contain various flavonoid compounds. Quercetin (5,7,3′,4′-tetrahydroflavone), a secondary metabolite in hops, has been proven to be directly mutagenic in the *Salmonella* strains TA98 and TA100.[16] Investigations of extracts of hops cultures will show if mutagenic activity can be correlated to the amount of quercetin in the plants. Furthermore, at the end of the vegetation period plant material is ploughed into the soil during tillage. To decide if mutagenic activity in agricultural soils may partly derive from the cultivated hops itself, mutagenicity tests with extracts of hops plants and extracts of soils collected at various seasons have to be performed.

As already mentioned, various studies reported detectable amounts of PAH in soils. Therefore, the PAH content in the soil samples was investigated. Figure 3 shows the comparison of an external standard with a soil extract of hops culture, where, in addition to the characterized PAH, a large number of unknown compounds was observed. Mutagenicity of the known PAH is indicated in Figure 3. The total PAH content in the soil samples varied from 33 to 1800 μg/kg soil as shown in Table 1. Soils with high mutagenic activity contained higher amounts of PAH than soils with low mutagenic activity. The highest

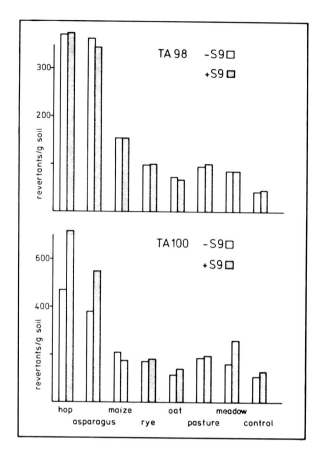

FIGURE 2.   Mutagenicity of soil extracts from various cultures using *Salmonella* strains TA98 and TA100 with and without S9 mix. Tests were performed with 1.25 mg S9 protein per plate of Clophen A50-activated rat liver and 2×10^8 bacteria per plate.

PAH content found in soils of hops cultures correlated with the highest number of induced revertants. Similar mutagenicity in TA98 (about 350 colonies per plate) was observed with 5 μg benzo[a]pyrene in the presence of S9 mix.

The PAH contents of the tested soil samples were, with one exception, in good agreement with data of Kunte[19] who reported that most agricultural soils (74%) contain 50 to 500 μg PAH per kilogram of soil. Thus, a distinct PAH content exists in all soils and may be caused by sedimentation of airborne particles.[20,21] It may contribute to the mutagenicity of soil extracts.

Table 1 compares data of the content of PAH and humus in the soils tested as well as the amount of nitrogen fertilizers and pesticides applied to the cultures. No correlation between PAH and humus content could be found. The tested soil extracts of meadow and pasture were derived from moory soils and contained high amounts of organic matter, but showed low amounts of PAH and also low mutagenicity.

The common nitrogen fertilizers were mixtures of ammonium or nitrate salts and calcium cyanamide which is simultaneously used as herbicide for asparagus cultures. Soil extracts of asparagus cultures showed 9-fold higher numbers of induced revertants than the control. This increased mutagenicity correlates with a high amount of nitrogen fertilizers applied as $[NH_4NO_3 + CaCO_3]$ which is transformed to the herbicide calcium cyanamide $[CaCN_2]$ in the presence of soil bacteria. Moreover, it is known that intensive fertilization enhances

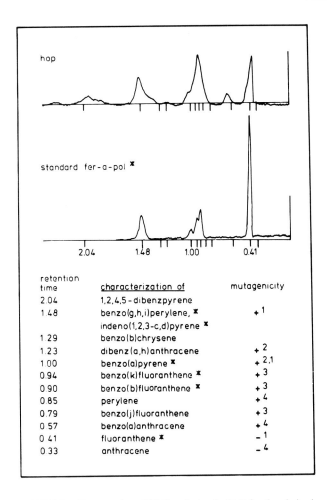

FIGURE 3. Reverse-phase HPLC analysis of a PAH fraction derived from an agricultural soil and of a PAH mixture (standard fer-a-pol). Chromatographic conditions: 160 × 5 mm LiChrosorb RP-18 column, 80:20 (v/v) $CH_3OH:H_2O$ flow rate 1 mℓ/min. Fluorescence detector: 325 nm excitation, >465 nm emission. Data on mutagenicity testing of the PAH have been obtained from the following papers 1 to 4 as indicated in the figure (Reference 1: Tokiwa et al.,[5] Reference 2: Andrews et al.,[17] Reference 3: Lavoie, 3rd Batelle Symp., Columbus. Ohio, 1978, and Reference 4: Purchase et al.[18]).

bacterial activity in soils. Thus, the conversion of nonmutagenic compounds to mutagenic derivatives may be considered as a source for the higher mutagenicity in soil of asparagus cultures.

The pesticides applied were organophosphorus (dimefox, methamidophos, omethoate, bromophos) and carbamate (methomyl, mercaptodimethur) insecticides and urea (methabenzthiazuron), and phenoxy acid (dichlorprop, 2,4,5-T, MCPA, MCCP) herbicides. Numerous reports on the mutagenicity of pesticides have been published[22,23] and there is no indication that these pesticides show mutagenic activity in the *Salmonella* strains. However, microbial and plant activity affect the persistence of the pesticides in the natural environment. Organophosphorus insecticides[24] are hydrolyzed to diesters of phosphoric acid and alcohols, thiols, or phenols. In microorganisms, phenoxy acid herbicides[25] are degraded completely to water, carbon dioxide, and chloride, whereas in plants metabolites are formed by decarboxylation, ring hydroxylation, and conjugation reactions. As yet, not much is known about

Table 1

COMPARISON OF PAH AND HUMUS CONTENT IN SOIL SAMPLES AND APPLICATION OF N-FERTILIZERS AND PESTICIDES

Soil of cultures	PAH (μg/g soil)	Humus (%)[a]	Fertilizer (kg/ha)[b]	Pesticide (kg/ha)
Hop	>1 (1.8)	2.79	558	0.15—4[c]
Asparagus	>0.1	1.86	1018	150[d]
Maize	>0.05	1.89	400	0.50—1[e]
Rye		1.98	282	0.40—3[f]
Pasture	>0.01	7.48	—	—
Meadow		12.04	338	—

[a] Percentage dry weight.
[b] Mixtures of [$(NH_4)_2SO_4$ + $(NH_4)_2HPO_4$], [NH_4NO_3 + $CaCO_3$], $CaCN_2$.
[c] Mixtures of dimefox-tetramethylphosphorodiamic fluoride, methamidophos-O,S-dimethyl phosphoroamidothioate, ome-thoate-O,O-dimethyl S-[2-(methlamino)-2-oxyethyl]phos-phorothioate, methomyl-methyl$N$-[[(methylamino)carbony]-oxy]ethanimidothioate.
[d] $CaCN_2$ and formation from [NH_4NO_3 + $CaCO_3$] with soil bacteria.
[e] Mixtures of mercaptodimethur-1,3-dimethyl-3-(2-benzthiazolyl) urea, atrazine-2-chloro-4-ethylamino-6-isopropylamino-s-tria-zine, bromophos-O-(4-bromo-2,5-dichlorphenyl)O,O-dimethyl phosphorothioate.
[f] Mixtures of methabenzthiazuron-N-2-benzothiazolyl-N,N-di-methylurea, dichlorprop-2-(2,4-dichlorophenoxy)propionic acid, 2,4,5-T-2,4,5-trichlorophenoxyacetic acid, MCPA-4-chloro-2-methylphenoxyacetic acid, MCPP-2-(4-chloro-2-methylphen-oxy) propionic acid.

the further fate and the properties of metabolites in plants and even less about the conditions required for bacterial degradation and transformation. These processes lead to the formation of numerous substances and may be another possible source for the mutagenic activity in agricultural soils.

IV. CONCLUDING REMARKS

Our investigations led to the conclusion that in all agricultural soils a distinct mutagenic activity exists which is increased in soils of special cultures (hops, asparagus). Moreover, PAH contents of the analyzed soil extracts correlate with the level of mutagenicity. The major source for this distinct mutagenicity may derive from sedimentation of mutagenic airborne particles. The significantly higher mutagenicity in soils of special cultures may derive from naturally occurring mutagens in the cultivated plants which are ploughed into the soil by intensive tillage. Moreover, soil microflora may convert nonmutagenic compounds to mu-tagenic derivatives. Characterization of the mutagenic substances may clarify which sources are responsible for the mutagenic activity in the various soil samples.

REFERENCES

1. **Van Kreijl, C. F., Kool, H. J., de Vries, M., van Kranen, H. J., and de Greef, E.,** Mutagenic activity in the rivers Rhine and Meuse in the Netherlands, *Sci. Total Environ.,* 15, 137, 1980.
2. **Heartlein, M. W., DeMarini, D. M., Katz, A. J., Means, J. C., Plewa, M. J., and Brockman, H. E.,** Mutagenicity of municipal water obtained from an agricultural area, *Environ. Mutagenesis,* 3, 519, 1981.
3. **Chrisp, C. E. and Fisher, G. L.,** Mutagenicity of airborne particles, *Mutat. Res.,* 76, 143, 1980.
4. **Grasso, P. and O'Hare, C.,** Carcinogens in food, in *Chemical Carcinogens,* Searle, C. E., Ed., American Chemical Society, Washington, D.C., 1976, chap. 14.
5. **Tokiwa, H., Morita, K., Takeyoshi, H., Takahashi, K., and Ohnishi, Y.,** Detection of mutagenic activity in particulate air pollutants, *Mutat. Res.,* 48, 237, 1977.
6. **Blumer, M.,** Benzpyrenes in soil, *Science,* 134, 474, 1961.
7. **Borneff, J. and Fischer, R.,** Kanzerogene Substanzen in Wasser und Boden. XI. Polyzyklische Aromatische Kohlenwasserstoffe in Walderde, *Arch. Hyg. Bakteriol.,* 146, 430, 1962.
8. **Shabad, L. M., Cohan, Y. L., Ilnitsky, A. P., Khesina, A. Y., Shcherbak, N. P., and Smirnov, G. A.,** The carcinogenic hydrocarbon benzo(a)pyrene in the soil, *J. Natl. Cancer Inst.,* 47, 1179, 1971.
9. **Blumer, M. and Youngblood, W. W.,** Polycyclic aromatic hydrocarbons in soils and recent sediments, *Science,* 188, 53, 1974.
10. **Springer, U. and Klee, J.,** Prüfung der Leistungsfähigkeit von einigen wichtigeren Verfahren zur Bestimmung des Kohlenstoffs mittels Chromschwefelsäure sowie Vorschlag einer neuen Schnellmethode, *Z. Pflanzenernaehr., Dueng. Bodenkd.,* 64, 1, 1954.
11. **Ames, B. N., McCann, J., and Yamasaki, E.,** Methods for detecting carcinogens and mutagens with the *Salmonella*/mammalian-microsome mutagenicity test, *Mutat. Res.,* 31, 347, 1975.
12. **Das, B. S. and Thomas, G. H.,** Fluorescence detection in high performance liquid chromatographic determination of polycyclic aromatic hydrocarbons, *Anal. Chem.,* 50, 967, 1978.
13. **Schoental, R.,** Carcinogens in plants and microorganisms, in *Chemical Carcinogens,* Searle, C. E., Ed., American Chemical Society, Washington, D.C., 1976, chap. 12.
14. **Brown, J. P., Dietrich, P. S., and Brown, R. J.,** Frameshift mutagenicity of certain naturally occurring phenolic compounds in the *Salmonella*/microsome test: activation of anthraquinone and flavonol glycosides by gut bacterial enzymes, *Biochem. Soc. Trans.,* 5, 1489, 1977.
15. **Hashimoto, Y., Shudo, K., Okamoto, T., Nagao, M., Takahashi, Y., and Sugimura, T.,** Mutagenicities of 4-hydroxy-1,4-benzoxazinones naturally occurring in maize plants and of related compounds, *Mutat. Res.,* 66, 191, 1979.
16. **Bjeldanes, L. F. and Chang, G. W.,** Mutagenic activity of quercetin and related compounds, *Science,* 197, 577, 1977.
17. **Andrews, A. W., Thibault, L. H., and Lijinsky, W.,** The relationship between carcinogenicity and mutagenicity of some polynuclear hydrocarbons, *Mutat. Res.,* 51, 311, 1978.
18. **Purchase, I. F. H., Longstaff, E., Ashby, J., Styles, J. A., Anderson, D., Lefevre, P. A., and Westwood, F. R.,** An evaluation of 6 short-term tests for detecting organic chemical carcinogens, *Br. J. Cancer,* 37, 873, 1978.
19. **Kunte, H.,** Polycyclic aromatic hydrocarbons in agricultural soil, *Zentralbl. Bakteriol. Hyg.,* 164, 469, 1977.
20. **Wang, C. Y., Lee, M., King, C. M., and Warner, P. O.,** Evidence for nitroaromatics as direct-acting mutagens of airborne particulates, *Chemosphere,* 9, 83, 1980.
21. **Tokiwa, H., Kitamori, S., Takahashi, K., and Ohnishi, Y.,** Mutagenic and chemical assay of extracts of airborne particulates, *Mutat. Res.,* 77, 99, 1980.
22. **Shirasu, Y., Moriya, M., Kato, K., Furuhashi, A., and Kada, T.,** Mutagenicity screening of pesticides in the microbial system, *Mutat. Res.,* 40, 19, 1976.
23. **Andersen, K. J., Leighty, E. G., and Takahashi, M. T.,** Evaluation of herbicides for possible mutagenic properties, *J. Agric. Food Chem.,* 20, 649, 1972.
24. **Wild, D.,** Mutagenicity studies on organophosphorus insecticides, *Mutat. Res.,* 32, 133, 1975.
25. **Seiler, J. P.,** The genetic toxicology of phenoxy acids other than 2,4,5-T, *Mutat. Res.,* 55, 197, 1978.

Index

INDEX